Grade 8

This book is for Jean

Other books by Richard B. Lyttle:

POLAR FRONTIERS
HOW TO BEAT THE HIGH COST OF SAILING
A YEAR IN THE MINORS
THE COMPLETE BEGINNER'S GUIDE TO BICYCLING
THE COMPLETE BEGINNER'S GUIDE TO BACKPACKING
BASIC HOCKEY STRATEGY
PAINTS, INKS, AND DYES
CHALLENGED BY HANDICAP
SOCCER FEVER: A YEAR WITH THE SAN JOSE
   EARTHQUAKES
ARCHIE GRIFFIN (*with Edward F. Dolan*)
BOBBY CLARKE (*with Edward F. Dolan*)
MARTINA NAVRATILOVA (*with Edward F. Dolan*)

The Complete Beginner's Guide to Physical Fitness

RICHARD B. LYTTLE

Doubleday & Company, Inc.   Garden City, New York

Library of Congress Cataloging in Publication Data

Lyttle, Richard B.
  The complete beginner's guide to physical fitness.

  Includes index.
  1. Exercise. 2. Physical fitness. I. Title.
RA781.L9 613.7
ISBN 0-385-12773-1 Trade
    0-385-12774-x Prebound
Library of Congress Catalog Card Number 77–80896

Copyright © 1978 by Richard B. Lyttle
Printed in the United States of America
All Rights Reserved
First Edition

Contents

Preface … vii

1. Introducing Exercise … 1

Part One   *Body Talk*
2. Knowing Your Body … 19
3. Feeding Your Body … 28
4. Testing Your Body … 37

Part Two   *The Big Three*
5. Pliometrics … 49
6. Miometrics … 70
7. Aerobics … 83

Part Three   *Supplementals*
8. Stretch with Yoga … 99
9. Isometrics … 115
10. Weights … 127
11. Special Problems … 136

Index … 147

Preface

Use common sense about health and exercise. If you have a cold or a fever, don't exercise. If you have a chronic health problem, see a doctor before you begin any workout.

It's true that exercise programs can cure or control many problems, ranging from minor backaches to serious heart ailments, but these must be special programs, planned and approved by a doctor who has full knowledge of your particular problem.

If you do have a medical problem, the chances are good that you should be exercising, but your doctor is the only one who can tell you which specific exercises you should do and which you should avoid.

A few more precautions: If you are over thirty-five, have a complete medical check-up before you do aerobic exercises. And if, during any exercises, you experience sharp pains, dizziness, or any other unusual discomfort, go to your doctor.

Now, let's get started.

1   *Introducing Exercise*

Exercise is the key to fitness.

Ample rest and nutritious food are necessary for a healthy life, but exercise adds the zest for life. It's the frosting on the cake. It doesn't just make you live longer. It makes you *want* to live longer.

It's fun. It's non-competitive. It's free.

Furthermore, if the cautions in the Preface do not apply to you, you can start right now. So empty your pockets, kick off your shoes, and begin.

STRETCHING

Your daily exercise program should have three phases—warm-ups, vigorous aerobic activity, and cool-offs. You should spend about six to eight minutes warming up, from ten to thirty minutes at your aerobic workout, and a minute or two cooling off. Your warm-ups should provide plenty of body motion that will flex and stretch your muscles. You should begin with stretching exercises.

The Bend. Stand with your feet about a foot apart and your arms above your head. Bend forward slowly from the waist, letting the weight of your arms, head, and trunk pull you down. Try to touch

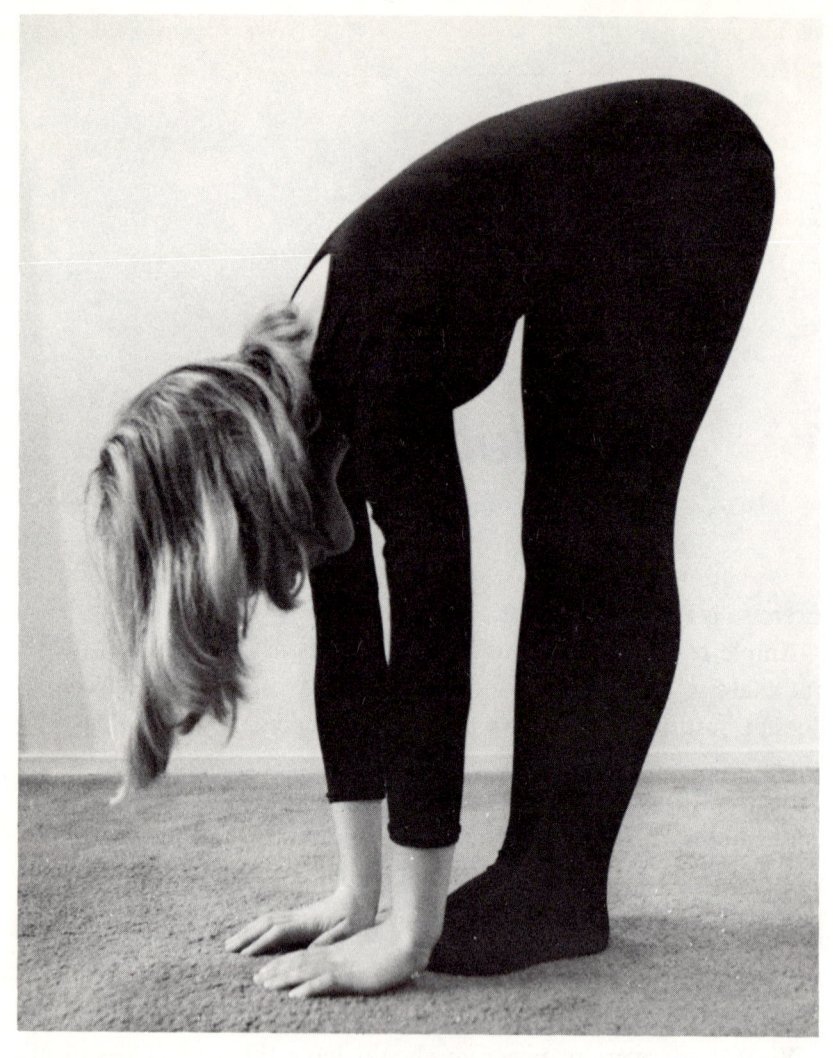

2 THE COMPLETE BEGINNER'S GUIDE TO PHYSICAL FITNESS

The bend is basic for flexibility. Don't worry if you can't touch your toes at first. Keep working at the exercise, and you will soon be able to touch the floor with your knuckles or your palms.

the floor between your feet. You may bend your knees slightly at first, and even so, you may still not be able to touch the floor. Don't worry about it. Your lack of flexibility simply points up a need for this exercise.

When you have reached your lowest point, straighten up, raising your arms high again. Then bend down once more, bobbing to

INTRODUCING EXERCISE 3

reach your lowest point with full stretch. You should feel a tug along the back of your legs. Do several bends, but stop at the first hint of strain or fatigue.

The Cobra. Lie prone and place your palms on the floor under your shoulders with your fingers pointing forward. Now lift your head as you straighten your elbows. Let your spine bend backward as your upper trunk rises. Straighten your arms as much as you can

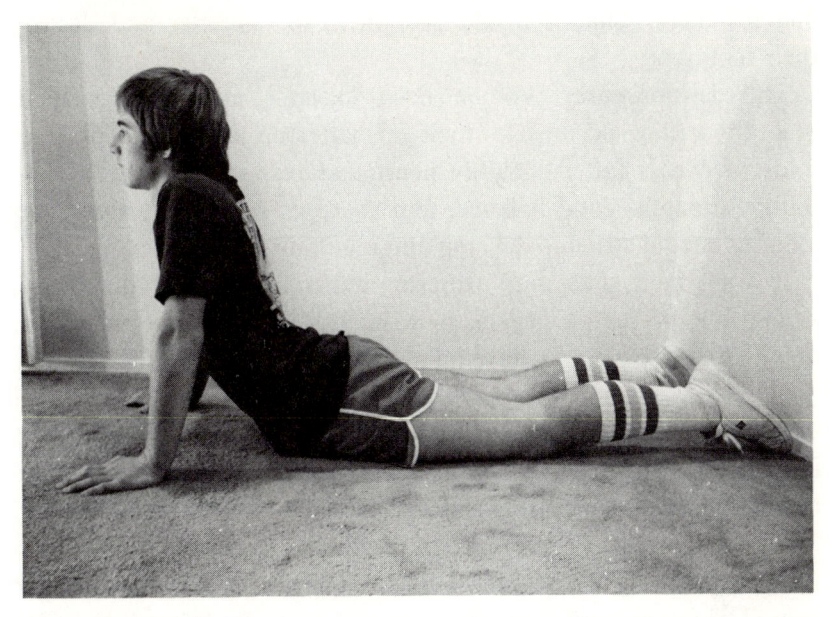

The cobra, a Yoga exercise, gives the spine backward flexibility. Hold the position for a count of ten and repeat at least once again.

without lifting your hips from the floor. Hold the position for ten seconds. (Counting one chimpanzee, two chimpanzees, three chimpanzees is a good way to count off the seconds.) Ease yourself back to the floor, rest a moment, and repeat.

This classic Yoga exercise is extremely valuable in giving the spine backward flexibility, something that is neglected in most conventional exercises. Don't worry if you cannot straighten your elbows fully when you begin. There is really no such thing as failure in any exercise. If you do your best each time, you are bound to improve.

A BREATHER

Since you should work into exercise gradually, take a breather and consider one of the major misconceptions about exercise.

For many years, girls and women were told that exercise was bad for them. That it would give them big muscles and destroy their femininity.

This is nonsense. Women need exercise as much as men. Smooth, well-toned muscles look far better on anyone's body than folds of excess fat. A healthy heart and respiratory system, flexibility, strength, good balance, and sharp co-ordination are things all of us should strive to develop and maintain.

It was once said that exercise and sports would damage a woman's reproductive organs. Now we know that women who keep fit with exercise actually have an easier time in childbirth.

Of course, none of this is to say that men and women have equal capacity and ability. Forty per cent of an adult male's body weight is muscle. Just 30 per cent of an adult woman's body is muscle. Men, thus, are generally stronger, but women are more flexible. They have less muscle tissue to restrict their movements.

The stretching exercises should be easier for women than for men. The following flexing exercises will be easier for men than for women.

FLEXING

Sit-ups. Lie on your back with your arms at your sides. Bending at the waist, come up to a sitting position. Lean forward as far as you can without bending your knees. Then ease your trunk back to the floor. Repeat as often as possible, but again, stop at the first hint of strain.

There are many forms of this exercise. You should include at least one form in your daily routine to give the abdominal muscles good strength and give yourself good health, posture, and good looks.

INTRODUCING EXERCISE 5

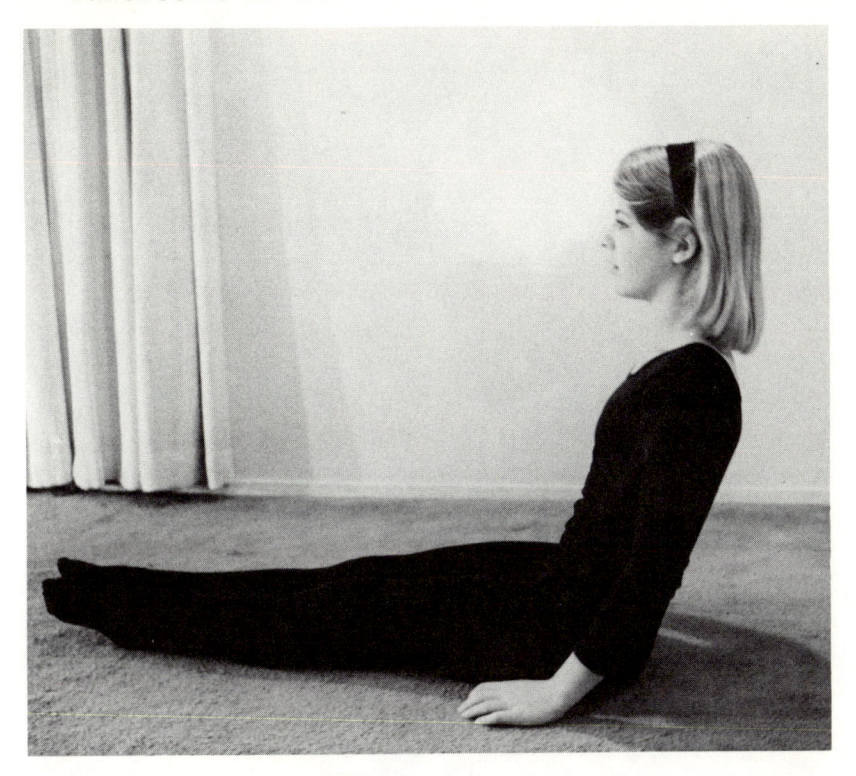

Sit-ups in any form will strengthen the abdominal muscles. This is the easiest way to do the exercise, but if you can't manage it, start with head and shoulder curls.

To increase the difficulty, do your sit-ups with your hands clasped behind your neck.

Sit-ups with knees bent will give the abdominal muscles even more flex. You will probably have to brace your feet under a heavy piece of furniture to do sit-ups in this manner.

For futher variation, use a curling motion to bring your trunk erect. First lift your head, then your shoulders, and finally the rest of your back. Lower yourself by reversing the curl.

Push-ups. Lie prone (face down) with your palms on the floor just outside your shoulders, fingers pointing forward. Keeping your body stiff, straighten your arms. Your weight should be resting on your arms and your toes. Now lower your body until your chest or chin just touches the floor and push up again.

That's the conventional push-up. It requires well-developed chest,

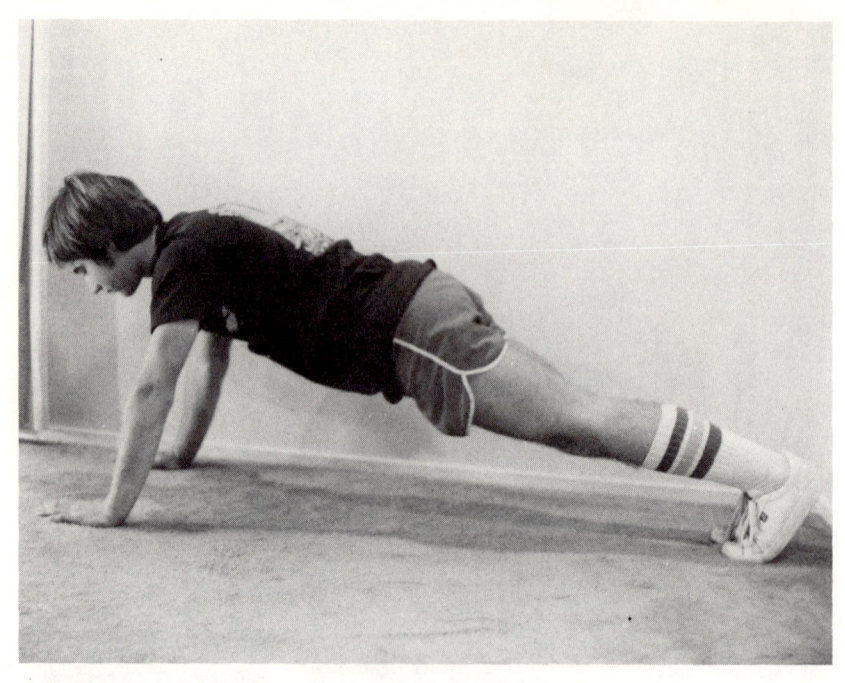

The conventional push-up is excellent for strengthening arm and shoulder muscles. Try to include some form of push-up in your daily routine.

shoulder, and arm muscles. If you are out of condition, overweight, or still going through spurts of growth, you may not be able to do a conventional push-up. There are many easier variations.

Instead of stiffening your body to your toes, stiffen it just to the knees. Push up with your weight on your hands and your knees. Girls and women often start doing push-ups in this manner, and don't worry if you are not able to advance to the conventional exercise. You will get plenty of benefit from knee push-ups.

If at first you are unable to do knee push-ups, stand facing a wall. You can begin about arm-length away. With feet together, lean forward, bracing your palms against the wall. Bend your elbows, but keep your body stiff. Let your forehead touch before you push yourself away. Eventually you can stand farther away so that you have to push harder to bring yourself erect. After a few weeks of this, you should be able to progress to knee push-ups.

INTRODUCING EXERCISE 7

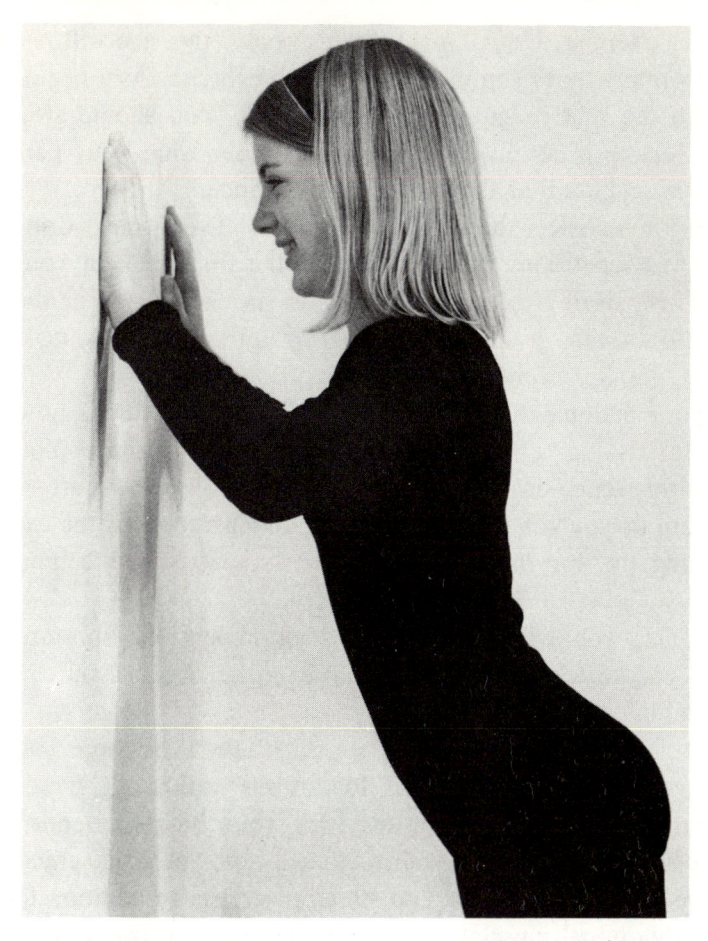

Wall push-aways are a preparation for push-ups.

ANOTHER BREATHER

So far, you have been introduced to just four basic exercises, but you have undoubtedly noticed already that much variety is possible. This allows you to pick the level of difficulty that fits your individual ability. Exercises with lots of variety also offer a step-by-step measure of progress. Once you can do several knee push-ups in succession, for instance, you can advance to conventional push-ups.

Another measure for progress is in the number of times you can perform each exercise. Unlike many fitness books, this one will not tell you how many times you must repeat each exercise. As a beginner, you are the best judge of your limitations. You should stop at the first feeling of strain or fatigue. Remember what your performance was and use that as your base for advance.

Suppose, for instance, that you could do just five sit-ups. Continue with five repetitions each day during the first week of your program. Then, during the second week, do six each day. For the third week, do seven, gradually building up until you are doing a fair number, perhaps twenty, with ease.

This is your maintenance level. Increasing your repetitions now will have diminishing benefits. It might even lead to boredom. You can stick with twenty sit-ups daily, making them a regular part of your program or you can switch to a more difficult form of the exercise—sitting up, for instance, with your hands clasped behind your neck.

Chances are, you will have to cut back repetitions substantially when you switch to a more difficult exercise. Again, you can increase gradually, week by week.

Now let's look at the possibilities for substitution. Suppose you have reached a maintenance level for sit-ups with your hands behind your neck. Switch to sit-ups with your hands extended above your head and reach for your toes each time you come erect. This is a great combination flex and stretch exercise. In addition to flexing the abdominal muscles, you are getting most of the stretching benefits that you got from the bend.

You can thus reduce the number of bends or even eliminate them entirely on some days. You will find that other exercises allow similar substitutions. You can change your program from day to day or week to week to suit your needs or your inclinations.

This is why so many exercises and their variations are included in this book. The aim is to give you full opportunity to find a program that fits your level of conditioning and rate of progress, a program that will always be challenging and never become stale and tedious.

Now let's tackle an aerobic exercise—an exercise that will give your heart and lungs a good workout. You will be working on

INTRODUCING EXERCISE

stamina here. Men usually have more natural stamina than women, but there are exceptions.

STATIONARY RUNNING

Take rapid, running steps, lifting each foot at least four inches from the floor. Try for a vigorous jogging or running motion. Keep your head up and your shoulders back. Let your arms swing freely. Stay in the same spot.

It sounds easy, but it actually takes hard concentration to get the

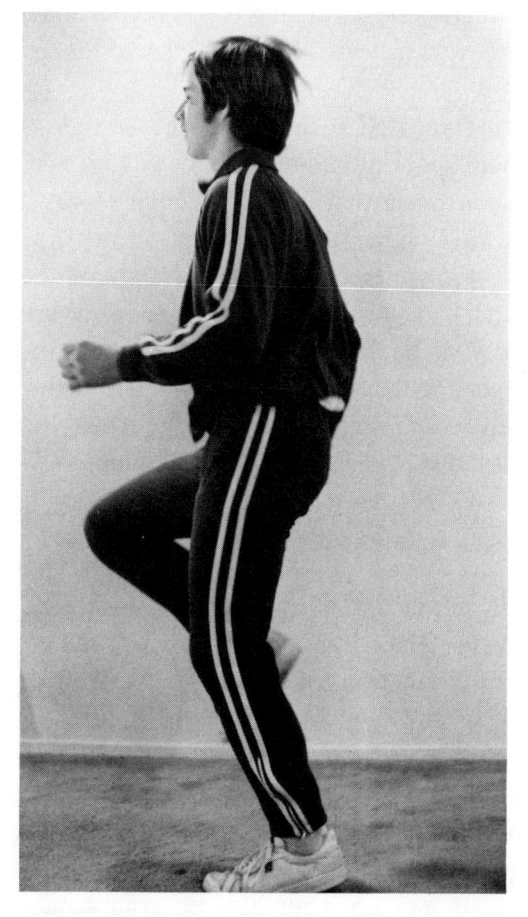

Stationary running will assure aerobic fitness in any weather. Lift your feet at least four inches with each step and let your arms swing freely.

maximum benefit from this exercise. Like other aerobic exercises, jogging or running in place must raise your pulse rate and your breathing rate to be of value.

If you are not in shape, and if you give this good effort, you will probably tire quickly. A minute may be your limit. That will probably be seventy to eighty steps. Each time you put your left foot down counts as a step.

Should this be your limit, stick with a minute of stationary running for the first week of your program. During the second week, extend the workout to a minute-and-a-half or two minutes. Set the pace of your progress to suit your ability, but do try to advance week by week. Eventually, if stationary running is to be your main aerobic workout, you must devote at least fifteen minutes to the exercise each day.

If you have trouble forcing yourself to lift your feet as high as four inches, pick an imaginary spot on the floor, a spot you hit with each foot. This will make you bring the lifting foot high to get it out of the other foot's downward path.

The chances are that you will prefer some other aerobic exercise such as skipping rope, regular jogging, running, cycling, swimming, or an active sport for your program. But you still should become a good in-place jogger. When weather keeps you indoors, when you're traveling, when you're pressed for time, or when you simply feel like doing nothing else, you can always jog in place.

COOLING OFF

Don't go abruptly from vigorous activity to complete inactivity. Aerobic exercise will concentrate blood in your legs, and it may take two or three minutes for circulation to stabilize. A sudden halt to activity can cause light-headedness, even a fainting spell.

You must include cooling-off exercises in your program. Stretching exercises that involve the entire body or walking with brisk arm motion will restore normal circulation. Perhaps the best cooling-off exercise, however, is the upside-down bicycle.

Lie on your back with your legs up, your hips on your hands, and your elbows braced on the floor. Now make circular motions with your feet as if you were turning the pedals of a bicycle.

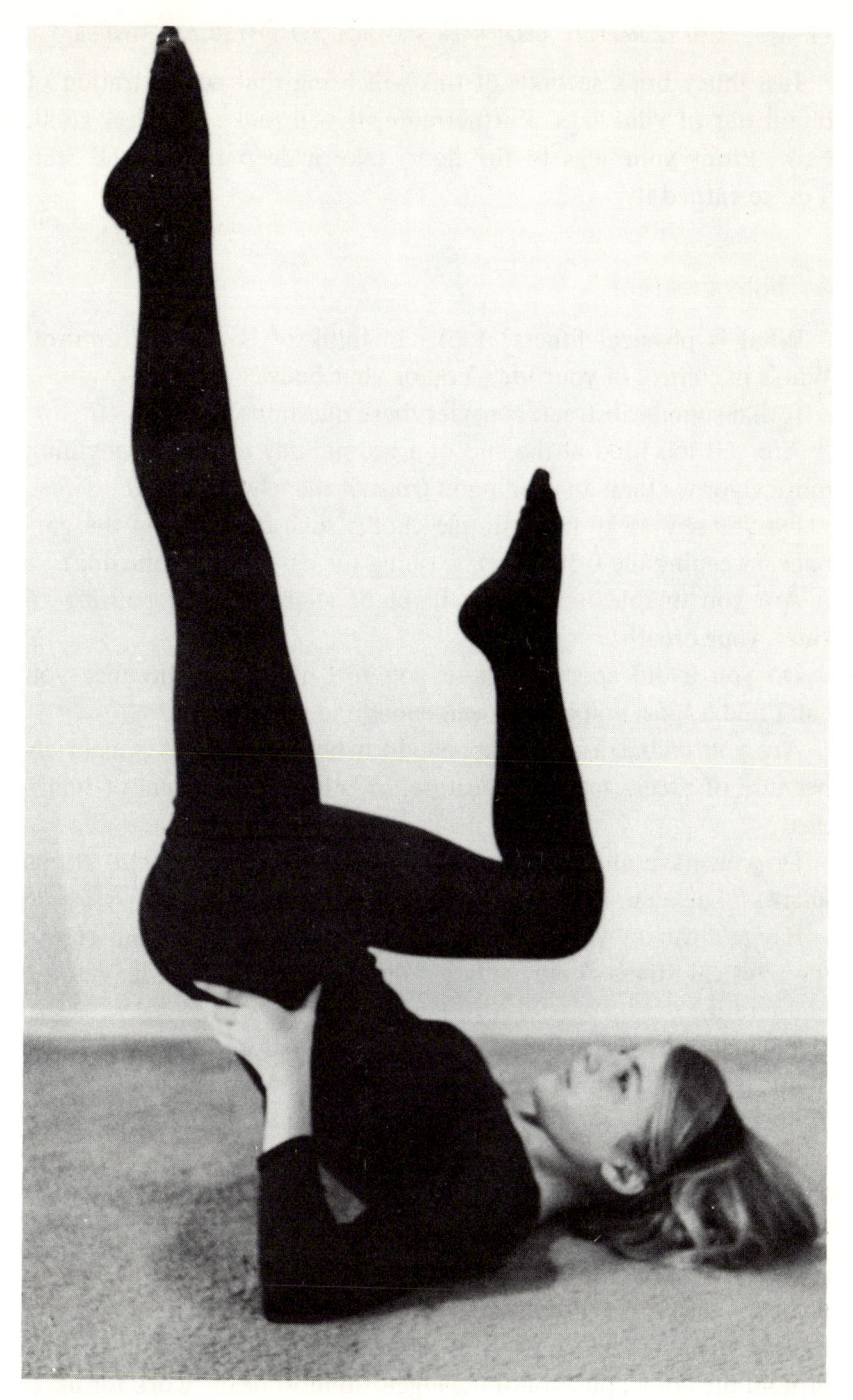

Upside-down bicycles, good for balance and co-ordination, also stimulate circulation. The exercise will fit well into the cooling-off phase of your program.

Just thirty brisk seconds of this will bring that concentration of blood out of your legs. Furthermore, it will make you feel good. Now, lower your legs to the floor, take a deep breath and rest. You've earned it.

BODY CONTROL

What is physical fitness? I like to think of it as body control. Who's in control of your life? You or your body?

If that sounds abstract, consider these questions.

Are you too tired at the end of a normal day to handle anything more vigorous than an evening in front of the television set?

Do you shy away from simple chores such as dumping the garbage, sweeping the front steps, washing the car, walking the dog?

Are you unable to climb a flight of stairs without pausing to catch your breath?

Do you avoid sports because you tire quickly or because you can't find a sport you can do well enough to enjoy?

Are you embarrassed to appear in a bathing suit or gym briefs because of excess fat, poor posture, or other defects, real or imagined?

Do you have chronic complaints such as poor digestion, sleeplessness, backaches?

If you must say yes to any of these questions, you are not enjoying physical fitness. Your body is running your life or at least some phase of it.

This situation is contrary to nature, but nature can do nothing about it without your help. In fact, if you don't take steps to gain control of your body, the situation will only grow worse as you get older. Even if none of the above questions seem to apply to you right now, the chances are, if you follow typical life patterns, that they soon will.

All of us, even when we are in good physical condition, tend to neglect our bodies. Modern technology practically urges neglect. Automobiles transport us. Elevators and escalators lift us. And around the home, push-button gadgets do most of the work for us.

Disuse of muscles makes them flabby or else stiffens them with

INTRODUCING EXERCISE

tension. We become weak and inflexible. Our lung capacity diminishes. Our hearts, the body's most vital muscle, cannot cope with extra exertion or excitement. We become slaves to our physical limitations. In short, we are controlled by our bodies.

Physical fitness will turn all this around. It will put us in control of our bodies. And we can gain and maintain that control through exercise.

DOWN IN HISTORY

Historically, exercise has received some bad reversals. Formal exercise came to the United States as calisthenics, a program that was developed by landowners in Sweden who believed the peasants there ought to look more like soldiers and less like farmers.

The military inspiration for calisthenics made them appeal to our Army and Navy. Everyone who has been through basic training from World War I on has had a full dose of exercise by the numbers. This achieved one thing—it turned people against exercise.

Early physical education instructors did not help. They believed that making large groups perform together in unison was the easiest way to handle the "problem students," those who could not make the team.

Often the instructors believed that exercise, to be of any value, should reduce students to an exhausted state. Needless to say, this attitude did nothing to make exercise popular.

Fortunately, thinking has changed in recent years. For one thing, doctors have discovered that exercise is good medicine. Exercise is now almost universally used in the recovery program for heart patients, and exercise is prescribed for many other disorders as well, including certain ulcers, arthritis, backache, insomnia, nervous tension, and indigestion.

Furthermore, it has been found that exercises need not be done in military fashion, that value is not measured by exhaustion, and that people can get enjoyment as well as benefit by exercising at their own pace, outdoors or in their homes, and without some gym instructor blowing a whistle or shouting out a cadence.

EXERCISE TYPES

Many new words have appeared with the new attitude toward exercise. They seem pretty fancy at first, and some of them are based on unfamiliar Greek words, but they are worth knowing simply because they are more precise than the all-embracing "calisthenics," a term, by the way, that has gone out of fashion.

Pliometrics. Exercises that lengthen or stretch muscles come under this heading. The bend is a good example of a pliometric exercise. Literally translated, pliometric means "more measure."

Miometrics. Exercises that flex muscles, such as sit-ups, to flex the adbominals, come under the miometric heading. Flexed muscles shorten, and the word literally means "less measure."

Aerobics. Exercises that boost pulse rate, such as jogging in place, qualify as aerobic exercises. Dr. Kenneth H. Cooper of the United States Air Force has pioneered most of the research in this field, developing a point system for rating the training effect or benefit of individual exercises.

These are the big three of any well-balanced exercise program. But there are also many other types of exercises, including Yoga, isometrics, and weight training, examples of which are included in this book.

Yoga. These exercises, many of them centuries old, originated in the Far East. There are thousands of different motions and positions but the Yoga given here is for stretching.

Isometrics. This covers exercises that call for flexing without motion. The opposite term is isotonics, flexing that produces motion. Isotonics is too general a term to be of much use, but isometrics covers a specific set of exercises. Clasping the hands at chest level and trying to pull them apart by flexing the arm and shoulder muscles is a typical isometric exercise. Isometrics will give you large muscles, but the value of developing muscles for size alone is now under serious debate.

Weight Training. Exercising with weights offers a good variation for your miometric or flexing exercises, but beginners must take great care to avoid strain or more serious damage to ligaments or tendons. You should not start lifting heavy weights without the close supervision of a weight-training specialist.

This book will describe standard exercises in all the above categories and conclude with exercises designed for specific problems or limitations. But before we begin taking up the exercises in detail, let's first take a look at the human body and its vital functions.

Part One　*Body Talk*

2 Knowing Your Body

Remember first of all that the body is made up of cells, millions of microscopic units, each with a specific design and a specific function. The cells form the tissues that make up systems. The diversity of work that cells perform is amazing.

Cells of glandular tissue turn out complex compounds needed for digestion, growth, and reproduction. Cells of some bone tissues provide the rigid framework for the body, while cells of other bone tissues make new blood. The cells of muscle tissues in the heart pump blood through the body. Other muscle tissue cells support the body's framework and give it motion. And the motion is controlled by cells of the nerve tissue, which send messages to and from the brain.

Cells also have the ability to reproduce themselves both for body growth and for the replacement of damaged or worn out cells.

Amazing as they are, however, the cells cannot function without lots of help. They need fuel, compounds produced by the digestive system and carried by the blood. And they need oxygen, also carried by the blood, to burn the fuel. This produces the necessary energy for the cells' remarkable work. It also produces waste which must be carried away by the blood stream.

Every cell in the body, thus, must be served with a healthy flow of blood.

The cells, the tissues, and the body systems are all interrelated like the parts of a delicate machine, a machine that can be easily thrown out of balance. But unlike a man-made machine, the body thrives on work. The more it works, the smoother it runs.

If injury or illness has ever forced you to stay in bed for several days at a time, you know what lack of work will do. Blood circulation slows down. Lung capacity declines. Muscles weaken. With prolonged bed rest, even the bones will soften or turn brittle.

On a smaller scale, this is what happens to a body that does not receive adequate exercise. Cell function declines. Tissues shrink and grow weak. Body systems respond slowly and inadequately.

We still don't understand fully how cells and tissues work, but we know enough about the body's systems to respect their needs. And just a brief look at the major systems is enough to show the importance of exercise.

THE RESPIRATORY SYSTEM

Your lungs are made of spongelike tissue that is both tough and pliant. The tissue is formed in two bags that hang inside the chest cavity. The lungs themselves have no muscles, but they expand and contract with the expansion and contraction of the chest cavity. As the rib cage and the diaphragm at the bottom of the cavity expand, air is drawn into the lungs, and as the rib cage and diaphragm contract, the air is forced out.

The strength of the muscles that control the chest cavity thus have a great deal to do with the capacity of the lungs. There is, however, another factor—the health of the lung tissue itself. It must remain pliant enough to respond to the chest cavity's changing size, and it must perform a remarkable gas-transfer job. The lung tissue absorbs oxygen for the blood to transfer to the cells and, at the same time, the tissue releases carbon dioxide and other waste gases that the blood has brought away from the cells.

The exchange takes place in alveoli, tiny pockets on the inside surface of the lungs. Each pocket is lined with thick webs of blood vessels. When these pockets become clogged or damaged, the lungs lose their efficiency.

Actually, the lungs never operate at full capacity. The expansion and contraction of the chest cavity is limited even in the healthiest body. The best anyone can do is about 75 per cent of full capacity. Most of us don't do that well, and the lungs of an inactive person might be performing at just 40 per cent of capacity. The actual performance is called "vital capacity," and it varies greatly from one individual to another. In addition, vital capacity must be considered with breathing rate—how much air the lungs can process in a fixed time period. This also varies greatly.

In his aerobic experiments, Dr. Kenneth H. Cooper found that a man in good condition could process as much as twenty times his vital capacity in a minute while a man in poor condition could process just half that amount.

Dr. Cooper's tests, however, showed a spectacular response to exercise. When those in poor condition participated in a program of vigorous jogging and running, their lung capacity soared. Many were able to double efficiency in just six weeks.

Polluted air will cut lung capacity. Smoke is particularly harmful. It carries chemicals that irritate—even destroy—lung tissue, and it also carries carbon monoxide, which blood cells absorb as readily as they absorb oxygen. Sending blood cells loaded with carbon monoxide instead of oxygen through the body is like shooting blanks. These blanks overload the heart, forcing it to pump faster to distribute sufficient oxygen. This is why tobacco smoking invites heart and circulatory ailments.

Cigarette smokers who inhale heavily may reduce their vital capacity by as much as 7 per cent. But again, Dr. Cooper found excellent response to exercise after the smokers kicked the habit.

THE CIRCULATORY SYSTEM

Blood has two specialized cell types. The white blood cells destroy germs while the red blood cells deliver fuel and oxygen and carry off wastes. The oxygen links with a compound in the red cells called hemoglobin. And a special enzyme must be present in the blood to bring this linkage about. The amount of hemoglobin and the controlling enzyme in the blood again varies with individuals, but barring disease, anyone who eats balanced meals can be assured of healthy blood with adequate oxygen-carrying capacity.

Of more concern is the efficiency of the system that circulates the blood—the heart, the arteries, the veins and the tiny feeder vessels that lead to and from the cells.

The heart is a muscle, and like all muscles of the body, it benefits from work. But unlike most of our muscles, the ones that wiggle our toes, lift our arms, or change our facial expression, the heart does not respond to direct messages from the brain. It is an involuntary muscle, working only as hard as it needs to work to meet the demands of the body cells.

As you sit here reading, try to make your heart beat faster. It won't work. The heart does not respond to such orders. We have to use an indirect method. We have to make the cells increase their demand for blood with fresh fuel and oxygen. We do this by exercise. When the cells work harder, the heart must work harder to meet the increased demand for blood.

A strong heart makes the blood surge through the body. Blood vessels are enlarged and made both strong and pliant. This, in turn, assures an adequate supply of fresh blood for all the cells of the body.

PULSE

Obviously, a strong heart and good circulation should be your first goals in fitness. The aerobic exercises, such as running and jogging in place, strengthen the heart by making it beat faster. The same exercises also benefit the respiratory system, stretch and flex select sets of muscles, and have many other benefits as well. But the best simple measure of benefit, or "training effect," of these exercises is your heart rate, or pulse. Specifically, you want to compare your minimum and adjusted maximum heart rates.

A young athlete in top condition will usually have a very slow minimum or resting pulse. The heart is so strong and the blood circulation so efficient that the body cells can be served adequately by a slow pulse. By the same token, the athlete's pulse does not soar dangerously high when he or she exercises vigorously.

KNOWING YOUR BODY

On the other hand, someone in poor condition might very well have a high resting pulse rate. Vigorous exercise will make the rate jump abruptly to a high level, perhaps a dangerously high level that will strain the heart or burst a blood vessel. This is why you must work into aerobic exercises very slowly if you are not now in good shape.

In some serious cases, anger or excitement will boost the pulse enough to strain a poorly conditioned circulatory system.

Along with conditioning, age and heredity also influence heart rate. There are no hard-and-fast rules saying what your normal pulse should be, but it can still tell you the training effect of your aerobic workouts.

First take your pulse at rest. You can feel your pulse either at the sides of the neck, behind the angle of your jaw or at your wrist at the base of your thumb. You will need a watch with a second hand. Make sure you have been inactive for at least five minutes before you take your pulse. Of course, you want to know the number of beats per minute, but you can take a short cut by using some convenient division of a minute. You can count the beats in twenty seconds, for instance, and multiply by three. Even counting the beats in a six-second span and multiplying by ten will usually give all the accuracy you need.

Your resting pulse may range anywhere from forty to ninety beats per minute. Whatever it is, jot it down and use your pencil to make some further calculations. Subtract your age from 220 to get your maximum pulse. If you are ten, for instance, your maximum pulse will be 210 beats per minute. If you are twenty, the maximum rate will be 200.

You will not reach the maximum rate in normal exercise. You don't need to. What you want is the effective rate, the rate that will benefit your heart and lungs.

To figure this, subtract your resting heart rate from your maximum. Then take 60 per cent of this difference and add it to your resting heart rate.

If you are twenty, for instance, and your resting pulse is 60, your effective pulse will be 144. You figure it like this: 220−20=200 (the maximum pulse rate); 200−60 (the resting pulse)=140; 60

per cent of 140 is 84, and adding this to 60 (the resting pulse again) gives 144.

Take another example using a ten-year-old with a resting pulse of 80. The effective pulse would be 158. It works out like this: 220−10=210; 210−80=130; 60 per cent of 130=78; 78+80=158.

Once you have done this figuring, you can experiment with jogging in place. You can find out how many jogging steps it takes for you to reach your effective pulse. Don't try to keep jogging while you take your pulse. The heart rate will stay up for a minute or so after you stop exercising.

If you are in poor shape, the chances are that you will reach your effective rate early, perhaps after no more than fifty steps. Don't worry if you are a few beats over or under the effective rate, but if your pulse soars well over what it should be, you should consult a doctor, preferably a heart specialist. It is not likely that you will have to give up your physical fitness program. Exercise can control many circulatory disorders, including high blood pressure and common heart murmur, but workouts in such cases must have a doctor's okay.

MUSCLES

Muscle is a tissue found in many systems of the body. The heart, as was mentioned, is a special type of muscle. The other types are the smooth muscles that line the intestines and other internal organs, and the skeletal muscles. The smooth muscles normally get plenty of work, performing their natural functions. Digestive muscles, however, can weaken if your diet includes nothing but soft foods and liquids. This is one reason why roughage, such as cabbage, lettuce, and grain products, is important in the diet.

Skeletal muscles, as the name implies, support and move the body's framework, or skeleton. In the past, muscle size was regarded as a measure of physical fitness, but we know now that tone is much more important than size.

Big muscles, in fact, can be a handicap. And if you exercise to build the size of your muscles without doing aerobic exercises that will increase circulation to serve the added tissue, you will lose muscle tone. The added tissue will not have a healthy blood flow.

A well-toned muscle responds quickly. It is ready to flex and stretch as required. It is not riddled with useless cells of fat and, while it is pliant when relaxed, it does not sag. But don't confuse tone with tension. Tension limits motion and slows response. Your stretching or pliometric exercises are designed to reduce tension.

Well-toned muscles assist the heart in moving blood through the body. There are no excess fat cells to slow circulation, and the flexing and relaxing of the tissue squeezes and opens blood vessels to stimulate circulation.

This is particularly important in removing waste products from muscle cells. When muscle cells work they produce lactic acid. For a time, lactic acid actually stimulates muscles so that oxygen-starved cells can continue working.

As the lactic acid builds up, however, the effect reverses. The acid becomes a poison in the cells. It halts cell function. Before long, the muscle tissue aches with fatigue and fails to respond. This serves as a safety valve. It prevents you from damaging cells by working them with inadequate supplies of fuel and oxygen.

Lactic acid has special significance for athletes, particularly runners and swimmers who must put on extra bursts of speed at the close of a race. During these sprints, the cells demand more fuel and oxygen than the circulatory system can provide, but the muscles keep working on the stimulation of lactic acid. If their muscles have a high tolerance against the poisoning effect of the acid, the athletes can make the stimulation last for several seconds, seconds that can be vital in winning a race.

Athletes thus train to increase their acid tolerance. They do this with anaerobic exercises such as hard sprinting. Anaerobic simply means "without oxygen."

Unless you are training for a specific sport that demands high lactic-acid tolerance, there is no need for anaerobics in your fitness program. Certainly, you should not take up anaerobics at the beginning of any program. Good lung capacity, a strong heart, healthy blood vessels, and well-toned muscles must come first.

During a normal program, however, you still may feel the

soreness and fatigue brought on by lactic-acid build-up in the muscles. This will fade away quickly soon after you stop exercising.

Muscle pulls and spasms are a different matter. They can cause several days of discomfort, and you should limit your exercises or stop them altogether until the pain goes away. If the pain persists, consult a doctor. Putting a strain on weak or sore muscles can tear tissues and cause serious damage.

Ligaments and tendons are part of the skeletal muscle system. Tendons are strong cords that connect the muscle to the bone. Ligaments are bands of tissue that surround joints and hold bones in place. Both tendons and ligaments can be torn by putting sudden demands on tense or poorly toned muscles. This is another good reason for beginning your exercise program gradually. It also stresses the importance of warm-up exercises at the start of any workout.

FAT

Some fat tissue is necessary in your body. It lines and cushions internal organs, and it forms an insulating layer under the skin which keeps your body from losing heat in cold weather and overheating in hot weather.

In prehistoric times, when people survived by hunting, fat cells also served to store energy. When no game could be had for several days, fat tissue supplied the energy necessary for survival. Then, when game was killed, the hunters and their families gorged themselves, storing up more energy in fat tissue. Some primitive tribes still live this way, but we don't. We eat regularly. Some of us eat too much, regularly, storing up fat we do not need.

This excess fat is unhealthy. The circulatory system must expand as our bodies expand with fat. The fat serves no purpose. It does no work. It is simply there, weighing us down, demanding service of the vital systems. Actually, volume for volume, muscle tissue weighs more than fat tissue, but muscle pays its way with work.

Excess fat invites circulatory disease because of the extra strain it puts on this system. Excess fat also makes any activity difficult, and the fatter we get, the less we feel like exercising. Furthermore, excess fat is unsightly. Fat people have a social problem, whether they like to admit it or not. Many fat people put on the pretense of being jolly, but psychiatrists have enough case histories in their files to tell you that this is false. Fatness does not lead to happiness.

It is still not clear why some people tend to get fat while others, with similar diet and activity, do not. Apparently some are simply born with more fat cells in their bodies than others. Metabolism also makes a difference. Metabolism involves the rates that our bodies use energy. Some nervous people are never still, even at rest they may be tapping a foot or swinging a leg. They use more energy than others. They stay lean when others grow fat. But metabolism does not fully explain the problem either. A combination of many different factors seems to be involved.

It used to be that fatness, particularly among young people, was blamed on glandular disorders. Today, however, this diagnosis is very rare. Glandular secretions are far more stable than once supposed.

We do know that excessive fatness can be cured with determination and effort. Obviously, it involves common sense about food. That's necessary for any fitness program.

3   *Feeding Your Body*

The right food is vital for fitness, but it's not always easy to know just what's right. There is so much nonsense voiced, written, and broadcast about food that it's possible to fall into a hopeless hash of confusion.

We can thank advertisers for much of the nonsense, but unfortunately some of it comes from so-called experts with pet theories, fad diets, or magic concoctions.

The United States Department of Agriculture does not dispense nonsense. Most of the information in this chapter, information that will guide you in selecting the proper foods for fitness, has been provided by the USDA.

First, however, let's consider a vital need that is not a food.

WATER

Water is needed for every body process and system. All cells contain water. By weight, 71 per cent of your body is water.

The body loses water daily through sweating, breathing, and excretion. The loss must be replaced. The body needs five to six pints of new water each day. The body creates some of this new water chemically when food is processed in the digestive system. The rest comes from water in the food itself and from liquids we drink.

FEEDING YOUR BODY

You should drink about three pints of water or water-based liquid a day. You can drink much more than that without doing any harm. The body simply gets rid of what it does not need. Getting too little water, however, can cause problems. One of the first symptoms of too little water is constipation. In most cases, constipation can be cured without any special laxatives. Just increase your daily water intake by two or three pints. That is far better than relying on laxatives, which can become a life-long habit.

Serious lack of water or rapid loss of water through sweating, vomiting, or diarrhea can cause dehydration, a dangerous condition. Early symptoms of dehydration are headache, weakness, fainting spells, and muscle cramps. Advanced dehydration causes death.

Remember, the body can survive for several days without food. It can hardly go a day without new water.

CALORIES

A calorie is a measure of energy. Technically, it is the amount of heat needed to raise the temperature of a kilogram of water one degree centigrade. All foods contain some calories, and the body is able to convert them into energy promptly or else store them until needed.

Even when you are sleeping, your body is using up some calories. As your activities increase, of course, you use more. Hence, a very active person burns up more calories than an inactive person.

Calorie need also varies with sex, age, and body size, but you can get a fair estimate of your daily needs by multiplying your body weight by fifteen. If you weigh 130 pounds, for instance, your food should provide 1,950 calories a day.

Since calories build body tissue as well as provide energy, we can put their effect in a simple formula:

$$\text{Calories} = \text{body tissue and/or energy.}$$

This is particularly important for weight watchers. As you can see, using up more energy through exercise can bring about a weight loss without any change in calorie intake. It is possible, thus, through exercise, to get rid of excess weight without going on a diet.

The following activities each burn up 100 calories:

> Seven minutes of hard running at 7.3 miles an hour.
> Nine minutes of cycling at thirteen miles an hour.
> Nine minutes of swimming at 45 yards a minute.
> Fourteen minutes of tennis (vigorous singles).
> Twenty minutes of golf, gardening, or brisk walking.
> Twenty-two minutes of bowling.

To put it another way, just a few minutes of activity is equal to one large pancake, two tablespoons of sugar, one five-ounce glass of milk, or one fried egg. Chapter 11 tells how to use the calorie formula to prepare a weight-reducing program.

Generally, fatty foods contain at least twice as many calories as proteins or carbohydrates. One gram of pure fat has nine calories while a gram of protein or carbohydrate contains about four calories. But there are several other significant differences in these three food types.

PROTEINS

A protein is a complex chemical compound containing many elements, including oxygen, hydrogen, carbon, and nitrogen, all of which are needed for the formation of amino acids. These acids, regarded as the genesis of life, are found in every cell. The variety of amino acids seems almost infinite, but in terms of body chemistry they fall into two separate categories.

Some acids can be manufactured within the body while others cannot and must be obtained from food. Those in the second group are thus called the vital amino acids. Proteins are rated according to the acids they contain, and the proteins containing vital acids get a high rating.

Since proteins are found in every organ, every tissue of the body, a protein deficiency is serious business. Glandular secretions that control muscle function, digestion, body growth, and reproduction all contain vital amino acids. Therefore fresh supplies of protein must be included in the food you eat.

Good protein sources include dairy products, fish, eggs, lean meat, and several plant products such as nuts, cereal grains, peas, and beans. Unfortunately, most of the plant sources do not carry an adequate supply of vital amino acids. This is of serious concern to vegetarians. They should at least include eggs or dairy products in their diets to be sure of an ample supply of the vital acids.

CARBOHYDRATES

Carbohydrates are produced by plants through a combination of carbon, hydrogen, and oxygen. The most common carbohydrates in our food are starch, sugar, and cellulose, all of which the body can convert to glucose, fructose, and galactose, compounds rich in energy that the body's cells require.

Carbohydrates are often called a quick energy source, while proteins are called slow energy source. The body makes more diverse use of proteins, and the chemical breakdown of proteins is indeed slower than it is for carbohydrates. But both eventually provide about the same amount of calories.

The body can manufacture its own carbohydrates from other food, but this process is possible only if a wide variety of nutrients are present. This is a very practical reason for a balanced diet.

Rich sources of carbohydrate are grain products such as rice, cereals, bread, noodles, root vegetables such as beets and potatoes, raw sugar, and other foods high in sugar content such as honey and sweet fruits. Alcohol, which is fermented sugar, is high in carbohydrate and calorie contents, a fact that weight watchers sometimes forget to their sorrow.

FATS

Just as some fatty tissue is necessary in the body, so are fatty foods necessary in the diet. Fats are compounds of hydrogen, carbon, and oxygen, which the body turns into fatty acids and glycerol, needed for several vital body functions, not the least of which is digestion.

Again, the body can manufacture some of these compounds, but others must come from food. And like proteins, there are an almost endless variety of fats. Chemists classify them by their bonding properties.

Saturated fats have all the hydrogen atoms bonded. They come mostly from animal sources and remain solid at room temperatures. One exception is coconut oil, a plant product, liquid at room temperature, but still a saturated fat.

Unsaturated fats, with some unbonded hydrogen, generally come from plants and are liquid at room temperature. Unsaturated fats, at the moment, are the most popular because the body does not convert them to cholesterol, a compound that gets in the blood stream and restricts or even blocks blood vessels. This problem is still under study, but doctors today almost universally order patients with high-cholesterol count to avoid butter, eggs, bacon, and other meats high in saturated fats.

All fats can cause problems because of their high calorie content. Too much fat will make you fat. As a general rule, your diet should be no more than a third fat.

VITAMINS

If our diets included plenty of fresh fruits, meats, and vegetables, we would not have to worry about getting enough vitamins. Actually, most of the highly processed foods today are fortified with vitamins. That's required by law. So there is a good deal of debate over the necessity of vitamin pills as a diet supplement.

The moderate view is that pregnant women, infants, those who suffer from prolonged illness, have chronic digestive disorders, or poor appetites should take vitamin pills. Healthy people who stick to balanced diets and have good appetites can probably do very well without vitamin supplements.

After all, human beings survived for centuries before vitamins were discovered. True, there were diseases, such as scurvy and rickets, that no one could explain until scientists began isolating these complex compounds.

Strictly speaking, vitamins are not food. They do not supply energy or go into building new tissue, but they are vital for specific body processes. A deficiency will slow down a process and cause fatigue, illness, or deformity. Strangely enough, some vitamins are

FEEDING YOUR BODY

toxic if you get too much of them. So it's not wise to stuff yourself with pills or a food rich in a specific vitamin. Don't get hooked by some vitamin fad. Let the medical researchers conduct the experiments.

Vitamins fall into two groups, those soluble in water and those soluble in fat.

The water-soluble vitamins, such as Vitamin C and those in the B group, while easy for the body to absorb, are not readily stored. Any excess is passed out by body excretions. Regular intake of foods containing water-soluble vitamins is thus important.

The fat-soluble group, including Viamins A, D, E, and K, are harder to absorb but more readily stored. This does not mean that one group is more important than the other. While the body can make several fats and proteins, it can synthesize just one vitamin—Vitamin D. So vitamins provide another strong argument for a well-balanced diet. Let's take a close look at some of them.

The B Group. There are at least eleven B vitamins that are vital, and there are several others that probably contribute to healthy bone marrow, skin, hair growth, and muscle function. A lack of B_1, a vitamin found in most cereal products, causes a disease of the nerve cells called beriberi. Lack of B_2, found in liver, nuts, and dairy products, causes the eyes to become hypersensitive to light. Lack of B_3 causes skin rash and diarrhea. Lack of B_6 causes nerve and muscle disorders. Lack of B_{12} causes anemia.

Vitamin C. Found in fresh fruits and vegetables, Vitamin C is necessary to prevent scurvy. Until mariners discovered the need of fresh produce for their crews, long voyages and explorations were dangerous at best. Vitamin C also assists the body in absorbing iron. It probably improves brain function, and it may prevent colds. But too much of it is toxic.

Vitamin D. Fish liver products, such as cod liver oil, are the only natural source for this fat-soluble vitamin. Lack of it produces rickets, a bone disease of growing children. Vitamin D is the one vitamin that the body can make, but only when the skin is exposed to plenty of sunlight. Today, most milk is fortified with Vitamin D. The chances are that you get an ample supply. Again, too much can be toxic.

Vitamin E. This comes from fresh whole grains. It helps circulation, is necessary for sexual reproduction, and may slow the aging process. As a medication, it is used to dissolve blood clots.

MINERALS

Unlike vitamins, minerals are simple elements or compounds, but they are just as necessary for specific body tissues and functions. Phosphorus and calcium, found in leafy vegetables and milk, are needed for strong bones and healthy teeth. Iodine is needed in the thyroid gland which controls growth. A few foods and sometimes natural water contain iodine. You can be assured of an adequate supply by using iodized salt.

Iron, contained in red meats, green vegetables, and sometimes in drinking water, is needed in the blood to carry oxygen. Iron deficiency causes anemia. Early symptoms are loss of skin color and fatigue. Lack of iron intake may be the cause, but usually anemia is brought on by the failure of the body to absorb available iron.

Mineral supplements are often needed, but don't experiment. A well-balanced diet should give you an ample supply. See a doctor before you start dosing yourself with minerals.

THE FOOD GROUPS

The USDA, in its long campaign for improved nutrition, recommends that Americans make sure to select foods from four specific categories—the milk group, the fruit and vegetable group, the meat group, and the bread and cereal group. There is a wide selection within each group, but the foods included in each are characterized by strength in specific nutrients.

The Milk Group. Dairy products are a good source of protein, fat, calcium, and Vitamins A, B_2, C, and D. Growing children should have at least three glasses of milk or the equivalent each day. Adults should have two glasses or the equivalent. The group generally rates high in calories. A glass of milk, for instance, packs 160 calories. Skimmed milk and buttermilk, however, have just ninety calories per glass.

FEEDING YOUR BODY

The Fruit and Vegetable Group. This group is strong in vitamins, particularly Vitamins B_1, B_2, and C. Minerals are also well represented. Spinach is one of the best sources of iron, a mineral that cannot be found in the milk group.

The group is high on protein and carbohydrate and low on fat. And even with the sweet fruits, the group is generally low in calories. A banana, a whole grapefruit, a peach, pear, apple, orange, and a glass of unsweetened fruit juice each contain just eighty calories. A cup measure of spinach, egg plant, celery, or tomato has just twenty calories. The group is high in water content and also provides roughage necessary for healthy digestion.

The USDA recommends at least four servings a day from this group, but it gives this warning. Overcooking can destroy many of the vitamins and other important chemicals.

The Meat Group. This is the big source of protein. The group is also strong in iron and many vitamins, particularly those in the B complex. Included are all animal flesh, eggs, and some plant products such as nuts, peas, and beans.

The calorie content of the meat group is generally high, mainly because of the fats that are included. Well-cooked lean meat, fish, and poultry will have up to 200 calories for each three-ounce serving. Other meats are higher. A hamburger patty has 230 calories, and a half cup of nut meat packs 400 calories. Four tablespoons of peanut butter has 380 calories.

The USDA recommends two servings a day from this group.

The Bread and Cereal Group. Generally rich in carbohydrates, this group provides quick energy foods that also deliver many vitamins and minerals and sometimes considerable protein. All grain and grain products, including rice, cooked and dried cereals, spaghetti, and noodles are in this group.

Many of the most valuable nutrients are in the skin or outer husk of grains which is often lost in milling. Flour from whole grain has more natural nutrients than the refined flour that is used in white bread and pastry.

The bread and cereal group has a fairly low calorie rating, but we often take these foods with fats or sweets that are high in calories. A slice of bread, for instance, has just 65 calories, but when we spread it with butter and jelly, we run the total up to 200 or more.

Pouring cream and sugar on cereal also makes the calorie total soar. A half cup of cooked cereal alone has 65 calories. A half cup of dry cereal has 110.

Junk Foods. The USDA does not recognize these in its list of recommended groups, but you should recognize them as something to avoid. Anything that packs a great many calories with few other valuable nutrients qualifies. Most candy bars and soft drinks are in this category. While they provide quick energy—something mountain climbers, soldiers, and athletes often need—they also dampen the appetite for more beneficial foods, something most of us don't need.

Few junk foods have much bulk. Indulgence often brings on digestive disorders. If you must nibble between meals, make sure that your snack has some nutritional value.

Although beer and wine have nutritional value, drinks made with distilled alcohol (hard liquor) definitely fall into the junk-food category.

4 *Testing Your Body*

You're probably curious about how you rate. It's a natural curiosity, but it's not the best reason for giving yourself a physical-fitness test.

The main thing you want from periodic testing is a measure of your progress. Your test score may point up weaknesses that will guide you in designing your program, but at the beginning especially you must not be too concerned about getting a high score.

The scoring methods are based on averages, and averages are misleading. You are an individual. There is no one else exactly like you. And don't forget, averages are not real people. They are just statistics.

Above all, don't turn testing into competition. You must not try to break records or beat the test scores of your friends. Your physical-fitness program is yours and yours alone. There are plenty of sports available to satisfy that need for competition.

Two tests are described in this chapter. The first has a simple pass-fail scoring method, and while it was designed for grade school youngsters, it will give any beginner an excellent indication of progress. The test does have some drawbacks. It does not measure endurance, speed, agility, balance, or co-ordination. Furthermore, it may be too easy for some of you.

If this is true in your case, use the second test. It was designed for boys and girls in their teens, but adults will have no trouble finding their scores by using the last column in the tables. Remember the scores themselves are not your chief concern. Your chief concern is how the scores improve between testing periods. In other words, your progress.

KRAUS-WEBER TEST

Developed by Dr. Hans Kraus and Dr. Sonja Weber, this measures minimum ability. The advantage over other tests is that anyone, no matter what age, can take it.

You do each of the following exercises just once and then go on to the next without stopping.

First Exercise. Lie on your back with your hands behind your neck, your feet together, and your legs straight. You may need a partner to hold your ankles firmly on the floor. Now roll up to a sitting position. Do not sit up with a stiff back, but lift your head, shoulders, and back so that your spine curls off the floor.

Second Exercise. This is much like the first exercise except you must have your knees bent with your feet flat on the floor. Again, you must curl up to a sitting position.

Third Exercise. Lie on your back with your hands behind your neck, your feet together, and your legs straight. Without bending your knees lift your legs so that your heels are at least ten inches off the floor. Hold them there for ten seconds. Then lower your legs. These three tests measure the strength of different sets of abdominal muscles.

Fourth Exercise. Lie face down with a pillow or blanket roll under your hips. Have a partner hold your ankles with one hand and place the other hand in the small of your back. Now, with your hands behind your head, lift your chest from the floor and hold the position for ten seconds.

Fifth Exercise. Starting in the same position, have a partner place one hand on your shoulders and the other in the small of your back. Without bending your knees, lift your feet off the floor and hold them up for ten seconds. The fourth and fifth tests measure the strength of muscles in your lower back.

TESTING YOUR BODY

Sixth Exercise. Stand erect with feet together and knees straight. Bend over and touch your toes with your fingertips. Don't try to extend your reach by bobbing. This test measures flexibility.

If you were unable to do just one of these exercises, your body is only in fair condition. Any failure or difficulty points to the area where you need work. If you passed all tests with ease, you can be pleased. More than half of the grade school children in the United States fail at least one exercise the first time they take this test.

YOUTH FITNESS TEST

Prepared by the President's Council on Physical Fitness, this was designed for boys and girls ten to seventeen years old. Those under ten should not take the test.

Those who are old enough should allow two days for the test. Do the first four exercises on the first day and the last three on the second day. And be sure to limber up with some stretching exercises before you begin on both days.

You must have a tape measure for some of the scoring, and you will need a stop watch that shows the seconds in tenths for the speed tests. You will also need a chinning bar, two small blocks of wood, and a soft ball.

Pull-ups for Boys. Grip a chining bar in both hands, palms facing forward. Your feet should be clear of the floor when your legs hang straight. Don't let your body or legs sway during the exercise. Pull yourself up until your chin is above the bar. Then let yourself down all the way so your arms are fully extended. Repeat as many times as possible, keeping count for your score on this table. It tells you the condition of your arm and shoulder muscles.

Pull-ups for Boys

	Age 10	*11*	*12*	*13*	*14*	*15*	*16*	*17*
Excellent	6	6	7	8	10	10	12	13
Good	3	4	4	5	6	7	9	10
Satisfactory	2	2	2	3	4	5	6	7
Poor	1	1	1	2	2	2	3	4

Pull-ups for Girls. This is done on a chinning bar that comes to shoulder level. Your feet do not leave the ground. Place them so

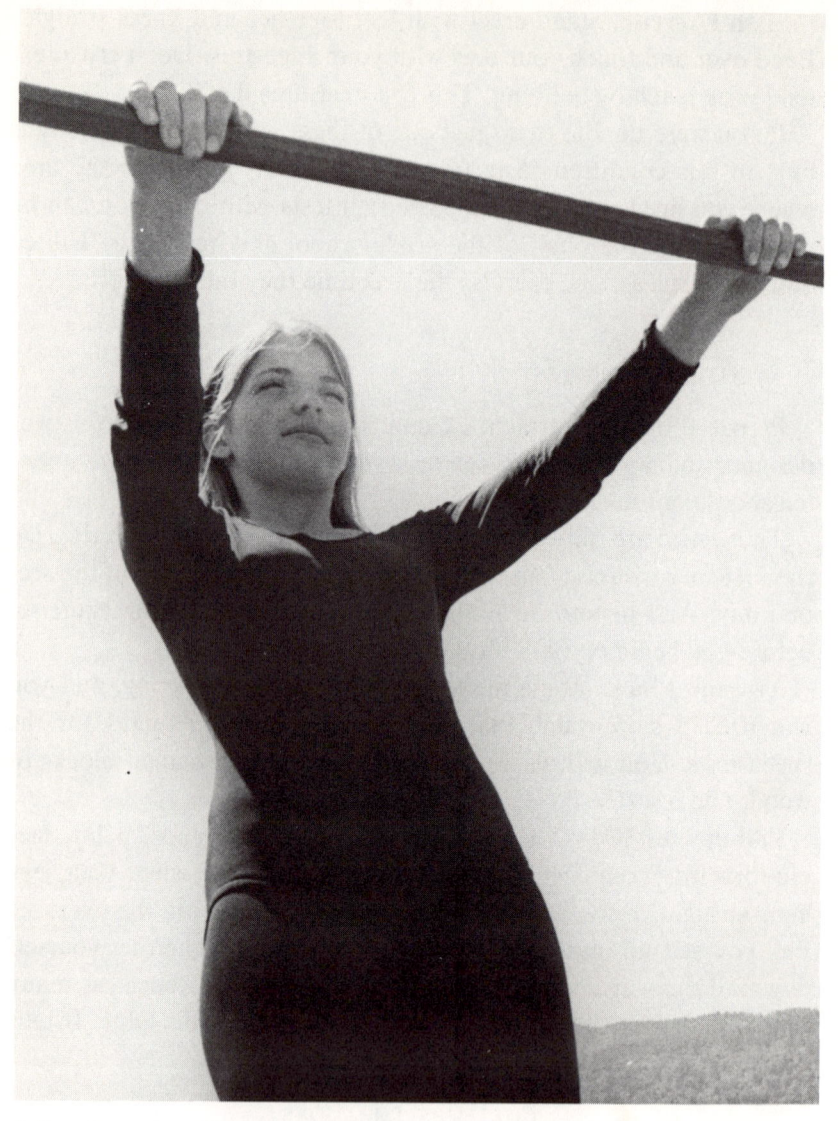

Pull-up for girls in Youth Fitness Test.

your heels are slightly forward of a vertical line from the bar. Keep your body rigid from heels to shoulders. Grip the bar with palms forward and pull yourself up until your chin touches the bar, then lean back until your arms are fully extended. Repeat as many times as possible, and keep track of the count in order to measure the condition of arms and shoulders on the following table.

Pull-ups for Girls

	Age 10	11	12	13	14	15	16	17
Excellent	45	45	45	45	45	45	45	45
Good	40	40	40	40	40	40	40	40
Satisfactory	30	30	29	30	29	22	25	25
Poor	17	20	20	20	19	12	14	15

Sit-ups for Boys and Girls. This is like the first exercise in the Kraus-Weber Test except that you touch a knee with the opposite elbow each time you sit up. Twist your trunk to touch your left knee with your right elbow. Then let yourself down and lift and twist the other way to touch your right knee with your left elbow. You will need a partner to hold your ankles. Each time you touch a knee counts as one performance. Do as many as you can WITHOUT straining, and use your count to figure the strength of your abdominal muscles on the following tables.

Sit-ups for Boys

	Age 10	11	12	13	14	15	16	17
Excellent	60	67	78	73	99	99	99	99
Good	47	50	51	54	60	60	73	63
Satisfactory	30	31	37	40	44	45	50	50
Poor	22	23	28	30	33	35	40	38

Sit-ups for Girls

	Age 10	11	12	13	14	15	16	17
Excellent	50	50	50	50	49	37	40	42
Good	33	34	30	30	28	26	27	25
Satisfactory	22	25	22	21	20	20	21	20
Poor	15	18	17	17	15	15	16	15

Standing Broad Jump for Boys and Girls. You will need a take-off line and a tape measure. Stand behind the take-off line with your feet about ten inches apart. Bend your knees, lean forward slightly, and swing your arms to give momentum to your jump. Take off from the balls of your feet with an explosive release of strength from your legs. Land without falling backward and measure the distance from your landing point in feet and inches from the starting line. Use the following tables, given in feet and inches, to measure the explosive muscle power of your legs.

Standing Broad Jump for Boys

	Age 10	11	12	13	14	15	16	17
Excellent	5'6"	5'10"	6'2"	6'8"	7'2"	7'8"	8'0"	8'4"
Good	5'0"	5'4"	5'8"	6'0"	6'7"	7'0"	7'3"	7'8"
Satisfactory	4'8"	5'0"	5'4"	5'8"	6'1"	6'5"	6'11"	7'2"
Poor	4'4"	4'7"	4'11"	5'2"	5'7"	5'11"	6'4"	6'8"

Standing Broad Jump for Girls

	Age 10	11	12	13	14	15	16	17
Excellent	5'4"	5'7"	5'8"	5'9"	6'0"	6'2"	6'5"	6'6"
Good	4'10"	5'0"	5'2"	5'4"	5'6"	5'6"	5'8"	5'10"
Satisfactory	4'5"	4'8"	4'9"	4'11"	5'0"	5'0"	5'2"	5'3"
Poor	4'1"	4'3"	4'5"	4'6"	4'7"	4'8"	4'10"	4'10"

Shuttle Run for Boys and Girls. Mark off two lines thirty feet apart and find two blocks of wood or other objects about the size and shape of blackboard erasers. Erasers themselves will work fine. You must also have a timer's stop watch and a partner to work it. Place the two blocks of wood beyond the far line and take a running posture behind the starting line. On your partner's signal of "Go," run as fast as you can to the far line, pick up one of the blocks and race back to place it behind the starting line. Then, without stopping, return for the other block and put it down beside the first one behind the starting line. Try this twice and take your fastest time (in seconds and tenths of seconds) to measure your flexibility, agility, and speed.

Shuttle Run for Boys

	Age 10	11	12	13	14	15	16	17
Excellent	10.3	10.4	10.0	9.7	9.4	9.3	9.1	9.0
Good	11.2	11.0	10.5	10.3	10.0	10.0	9.5	9.5
Satisfactory	11.9	11.6	11.1	10.8	10.5	10.4	10.0	10.0
Poor	12.3	12.0	11.7	11.5	11.0	10.9	10.5	10.6

TESTING YOUR BODY

Shuttle Run for Girls

	Age 10	11	12	13	14	15	16	17
Excellent	11.2	10.9	10.4	10.7	10.5	10.5	10.3	10.4
Good	11.8	11.6	11.3	11.3	11.2	11.0	11.0	10.8
Satisfactory	12.4	12.2	12.0	12.0	11.8	11.8	11.5	11.5
Poor	13.1	12.9	12.6	12.4	12.5	12.3	12.0	12.1

Sprint. This tests your speed over a course of exactly fifty yards from start to finish line. Your partner with a stop watch should stand at the finish line. Your signal to get ready on the starting line will be your partner's raised arm. He will start the watch the instant he lowers his arm. Of course, you must begin running then, full speed toward the finish line.

Your time in seconds and tenths of seconds will give you your score on the following tables:

Fifty-yard Sprint for Boys

	Age 10	11	12	13	14	15	16	17
Excellent	7.6	7.3	7.0	6.5	6.5	6.2	6.1	6.0
Good	8.1	7.9	7.5	7.2	7.0	6.7	6.4	6.3
Satisfactory	8.6	8.3	8.0	7.6	7.3	7.0	6.8	6.6
Poor	9.0	8.7	8.3	8.0	7.7	7.3	7.0	7.0

Fifty-yard Sprint for Girls

	Age 10	11	12	13	14	15	16	17
Excellent	8.0	7.5	7.2	7.4	7.3	7.4	7.1	7.3
Good	8.5	8.2	8.0	7.9	8.0	8.0	7.7	8.0
Satisfactory	8.9	8.6	8.4	8.2	8.3	8.3	8.2	8.4
Poor	9.5	9.0	9.0	8.8	8.8	8.9	8.6	8.9

Throwing Power. You need a standard soft ball, twelve inches in diameter, a tape measure, and a partner to assist you. Of course, you also need an open field or playground. All measurements are taken from a starting line, and you must not step over the line when making your throws. Take the longest of three throws to figure your score. If you do not have the use of a long tape, you can use a kite string or long cord and figure the length against a shorter measure.

Most effective throwing skill will be a wind up and run, starting six to ten feet behind the starting line. The following tables, with distance in feet, will give you your score for co-ordination and explosive arm power.

Throw for Boys

Age	10	11	12	13	14	15	16	17
Excellent	122'	130'	151'	171'	190'	207'	214'	231'
Good	103'	115'	132'	148'	163'	182'	190'	212'
Satisfactory	92'	103'	118'	129'	147'	164'	172'	185'
Poor	82'	94'	102'	115'	131'	150'	156'	167'

Throw for Girls

Age	10	11	12	13	14	15	16	17
Excellent	69'	88'	94'	106'	112'	117'	120'	120'
Good	56'	68'	78'	88'	89'	94'	99'	102'
Satisfactory	45'	56'	65'	75'	75'	80'	84'	86'
Poor	38'	48'	55'	63'	64'	67'	71'	72'

Six-hundred-yard Time. A measured track works best for this, but you can use any open space where you can mark off a distance of 600 yards. This does not have to be in a straight line. Remember, the bases in a standard baseball diamond are thirty yards apart. Five times around the bases will be 600 yards.

If you can run all the way, fine. But most people mix running and walking. The idea is to cover the distance in the least time possible without strain. The time in the tables below is given in minutes and seconds. An ordinary watch with a second hand is all you need to figure your score here.

This test rates your endurance, heart strength, lung capacity, and leg condition.

Six-hundred-yard Time for Boys

Age	10	11	12	13	14	15	16	17
Excellent	2:15	2:2	2:5	2:0	1:50	1:43	1:40	1:36
Good	2:30	2:24	2:19	2:13	2:5	1:59	1:51	1:51
Satisfactory	2:45	2:37	2:32	2:25	2:18	2:9	2:0	2:0
Poor	2:58	2:50	2:46	2:36	2:30	2:20	2:10	2:9

TESTING YOUR BODY

Six-hundred-yard Time for Girls

	Age 10	11	12	13	14	15	16	17
Excellent	2:30	2:25	2:22	2:24	2:20	2:27	2:23	2:30
Good	2:49	2:44	2:41	2:43	2:45	3:5	2:48	3:47
Satisfactory	3:6	3:1	3:3	3:0	3:5	3:6	3:5	3:4
Poor	3:21	3:16	3:21	3:20	3:21	3:24	3:23	3:19

KEEPING A RECORD

You will probably not want to take the full Youth Fitness Test more than once every six months, perhaps just once a year, but you can do individual exercises within the test to measure progress in needed areas more frequently.

Keep a record of your test scores. Your results and the date of the test can go into a notebook along with other data that will serve to mark your progress, including the increase in the number of repetitions of exercises in your fitness program itself.

Weight and body measurements should also be periodically entered in your notebook. If you are trying to gain or lose weight, you will want to get on the scales at least once a week. But don't neglect the tape measure. Remember, muscle tissue weighs more than fat. You might trim an inch off your waistline without changing your over-all body weight. This means you have replaced useless fat with healthy muscle tissue.

Those trying to lose weight should take regular measurement of the circumference of the thighs and upper arms, the abdomen at a point level with the navel, the waist at a point just above the hips, and around the buttocks at the fullest circumference.

Those trying to gain weight should check on the neck, upper arms, thighs, abdomen, and chest. Measure the chest with air partially exhaled from the lungs. The tape should be at nipple level.

In all measurements, keep the tape level and place it at the same points at each measuring to be sure of valid comparison.

Even if you are not concerned about too much or too little weight, regular measuring is an excellent way to keep track of your growth and fitness. Measuring forces you to take notice of body tissue. If the flesh around your thighs and upper arms is flappy, lacking in good tone, it's a good sign of needed work for these muscles.

Also, everyone can use a tape to get a good idea of vital lung capacity. Place the tape around your chest at nipple level and exhale all the air you can. Read the tape. Now inhale, expanding your chest as fully as possible. Read the tape again. The difference between these two measures is your capacity measure. A difference of less than an inch indicates a strong need for more aerobic exercise. A difference of four inches or more, on the other hand, will show that you have probably already achieved excellent aerobic fitness.

Part Two *The Big Three*

5   *Pliometrics*

The warm-up phase of your program should begin with pliometrics or stretching exercises, and you should select exercises with enough variety to give all parts of the body a good stretch.

This will not only make the exercises that follow easier to perform and more beneficial, but it will also protect you against muscle pulls. Furthermore, most pliometric exercises will stimulate your circulation and breathing rate. You will not sustain these exercises long enough to get the training effect of an aerobic exercise, but you will prepare your body for the demands of the more vigorous phase of your workout.

It must be noted here that there is rarely a sharp division between pliometrics and miometrics. Any body motion requires both flexing and stretching. In fact, your favorite warm-ups will probably be combination exercises that strike a fair balance between stretch and flex.

The descriptions that follow do not put such exercises in a special category, but you will be able to pick them out from the notations on side benefits. When a pliometric exercise, for instance, demands flexing of certain muscles, that will be pointed out. The descriptions will also make note of other side benefits such as balance, agility, co-ordination, and circulatory stimulation. In many cases, the variations for an exercise will increase such side benefits.

Don't be afraid to experiment on your own. That's part of the fun. When you discover variations for an exercise that increase its benefits and its pleasure, you will be particularly enthusiastic about that exercise.

Enthusiasm is important. We all have days when we just don't feel like exercising. It does not hurt to skip a day occasionally, but if you don't exercise for two or three days in a row, it may be hard to get started again. You will develop a sense of guilt, perhaps even a negative attitude about your whole program.

Having just one or two favorite exercises to perform is often all you need to break down any lethargy or negative attitude.

Beginners, however, must also be aware of too much enthusiasm. Too many start off with an overly ambitious program that can cause muscle strain or fatigue, two things that will kill enthusiasm in a hurry. Begin slowly. Don't take on too many repetitions of an exercise and, above all, don't try to do too many different exercises.

Your warm-up phase should include just five to eight pliometric and miometric exercises. They should encourage rhythm of motion, and they should be done in a sequence that will slowly increase the intensity of your effort.

The pliometric exercises here are grouped by the body areas affected and are generally arranged in increased order of difficulty or effort.

THE TRUNK

Reaching. Stand with your feet about shoulder-width apart and your arms at your sides. Lift your arms slowly. Keep them straight before you. When the backs of your hands are at eye level, come slowly up on the balls of your feet. Continue lifting your arms until they are straight overhead. Reach for an imaginary point far over your head. You should be up on your toes now with your fingers fully extended. Hold the position for a few seconds. Now slowly lower your arms and your heels to the starting position.

Actually, reaching will stretch muscles throughout the body, but you will probably feel most of the stretch in your upper trunk.

Balance is an important side benefit of this exercise. As your sense of balance improves, you will be able to hold the full exten-

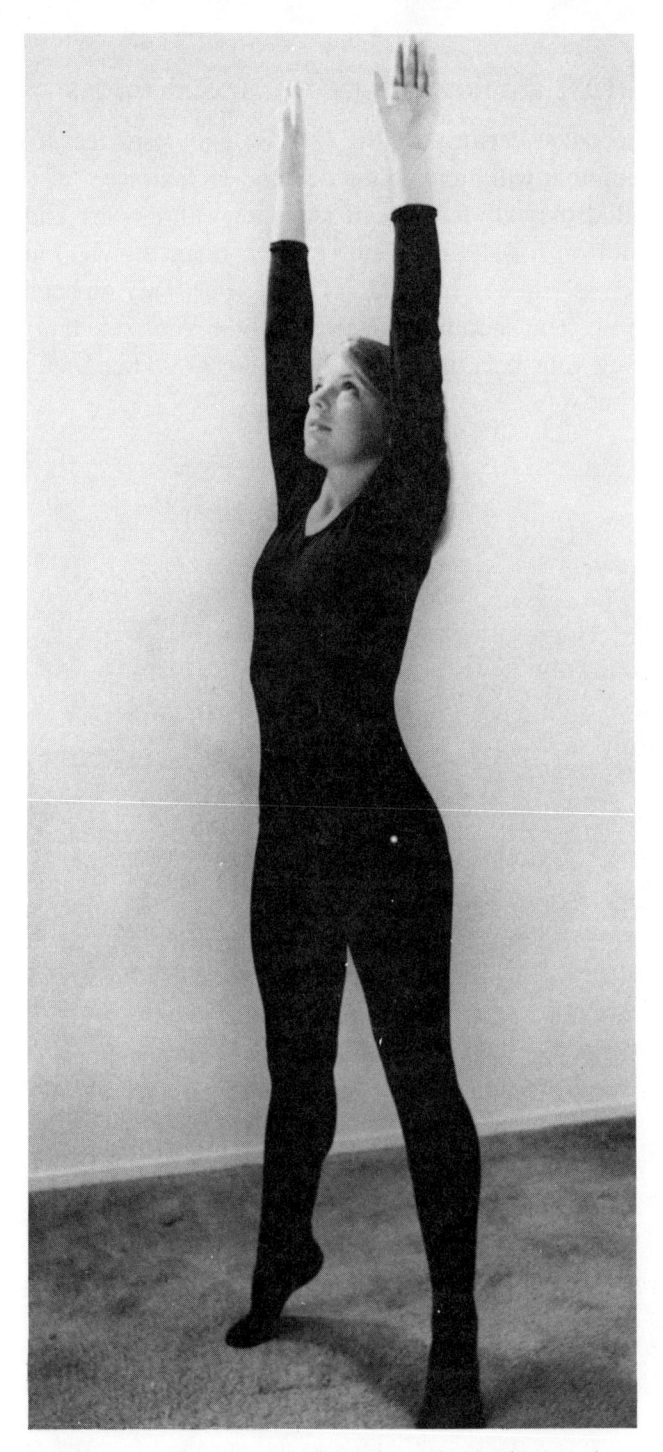

Reaching stretches muscles throughout the body, but the greatest stretch will be felt in the upper trunk. It is also good balance training. Eventually, you should be able to do the exercise with your feet together.

52 THE COMPLETE BEGINNER'S GUIDE TO PHYSICAL FITNESS

sion for several seconds. Performing the exercise with your feet together is a variation that will increase the demand on balance.

Swaying. Stand with your feet about shoulder-width apart and your hands on your hips. Bend from side to side. Begin slowly, but increase your pace as you continue. Don't twist your body or bend forward at the waist. You should feel a strong tug in your side muscles. You can bring your neck into play by leaning your head with the sway of your body.

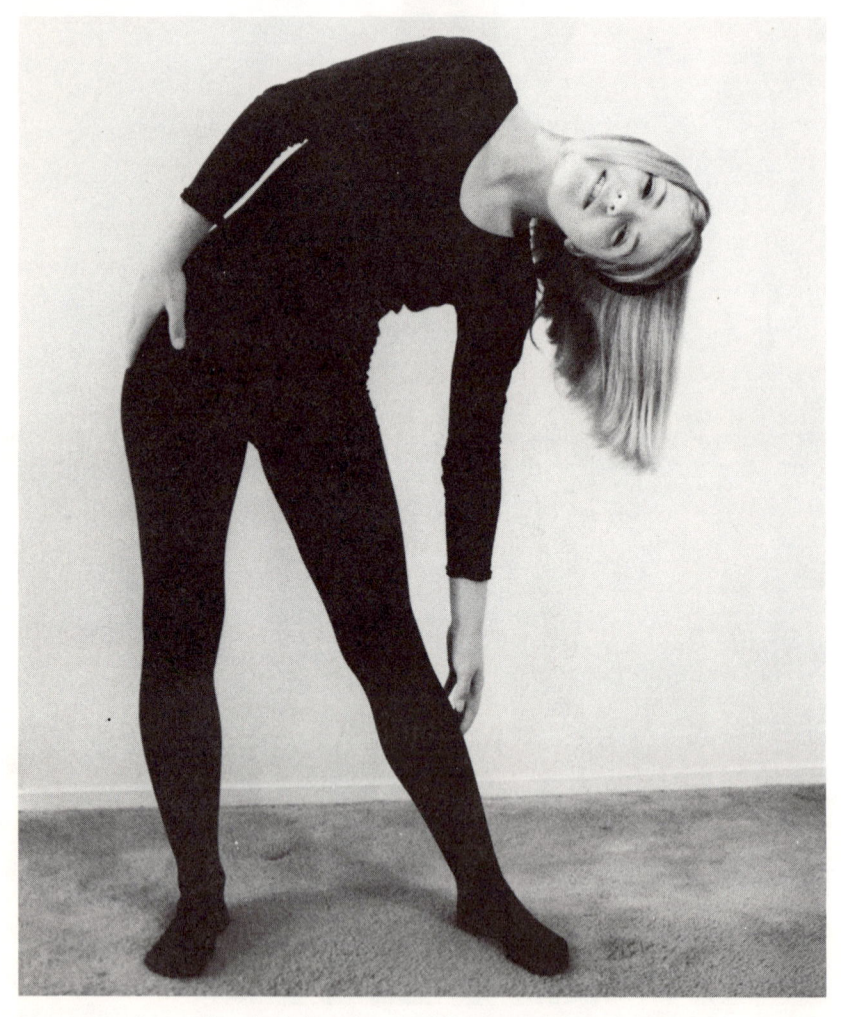

Swaying with your hands sliding down your legs will give the lateral trunk muscles a good stretch. Bob to reach as far down your calf as possible.

PLIOMETRICS

To increase the stretch of the side muscles, take your hands off your hips and let your arms hang straight. Now bob twice with each sway, trying to slide your fingertips well below your knees with each bob.

To extend the stretch to the muscles directly beneath your arms, do the sway with your arms aloft and your palms pressed together above your head. Your pace for this variation will be slow, but you will be giving your side muscles a good flex as well as a good stretch.

It is also possible to do the sway with your hands clasped behind

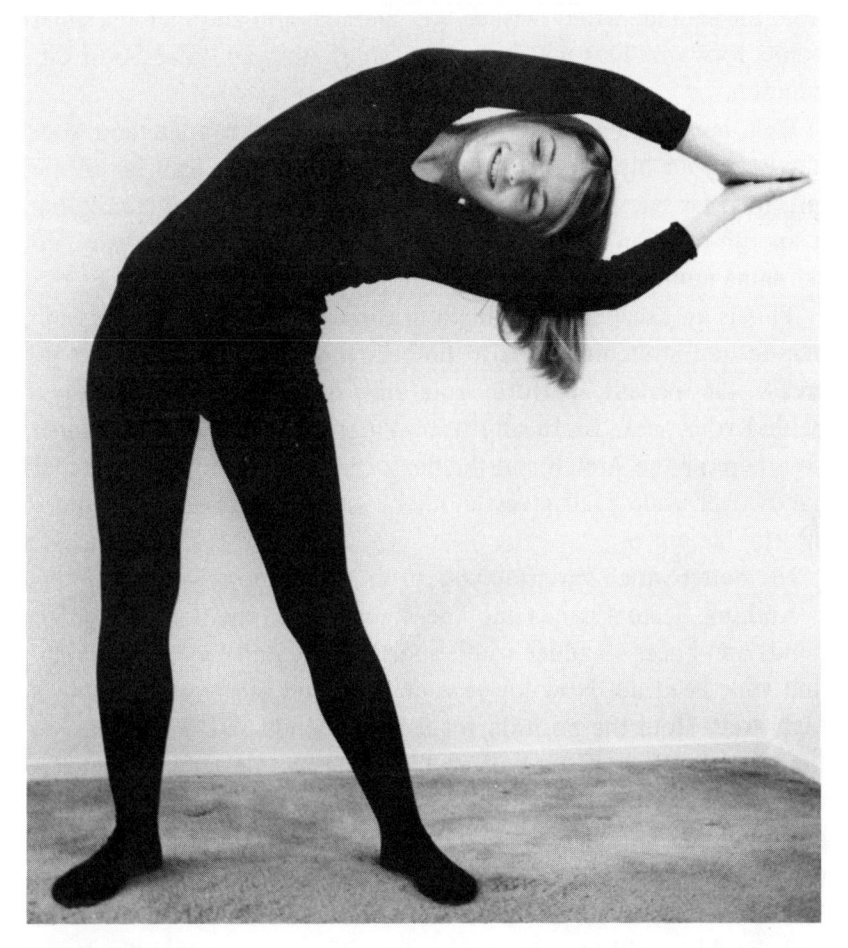

The advanced sway.

your neck, trying to bring your elbow as close to the hip as possible with each sway. The tendency with this variation, however, is to pull the head forward. This should be resisted.

Twisting. Stand with your feet shoulder-width apart and your hands on your hips. Twist your upper body as far to the left as possible and then as far to the right as possible. Don't bend forward at the waist and don't hunch your forward shoulder into your turn. This exercise will stretch a different set of side muscles, limber your hips and give some stretch and flex to leg muscles.

For a good variation on the exercise, extend your arms sideways from the shoulders and twist so that first one arm and then the other points forward. This will increase your rhythm and also boost circulation.

Rotations. Again with your feet shoulder-width apart and your hands at your hips, lean forward at the waist, then lean far to the left, then far back, then to the right and forward again, continuing a smooth rotation of the trunk. After several rotations this way, do the same number of repetitions in the reverse direction.

This is an excellent combination exercise in that it requires both flexing and stretching. It also limbers the spine and hips. To increase the benefit, perform rotations with your hands clasped behind your neck. By raising your center of gravity in this manner you increase the stretch and the flex of your muscles. Holding your hands over your head gives another variation requiring still more effort.

No matter which variation you select, do rotations slowly.

Arching. Take a hands and knees position on the floor with both hands and knees shoulder-width apart. Begin with the back straight and your head up. Now lower your head and raise your back in a high arch. Hold the position for a few seconds and then return to the starting stance. This limbers the spine and flexes and stretches the muscles in the lower back. The exercise also strengthens arm and shoulder muscles, and is therefore a good preparation for push-up exercises. In fact, if you have trouble doing push-ups at first, do arches in place of push-ups, for several days. Your arms and shoulders will soon be strong enough for the more difficult exercise.

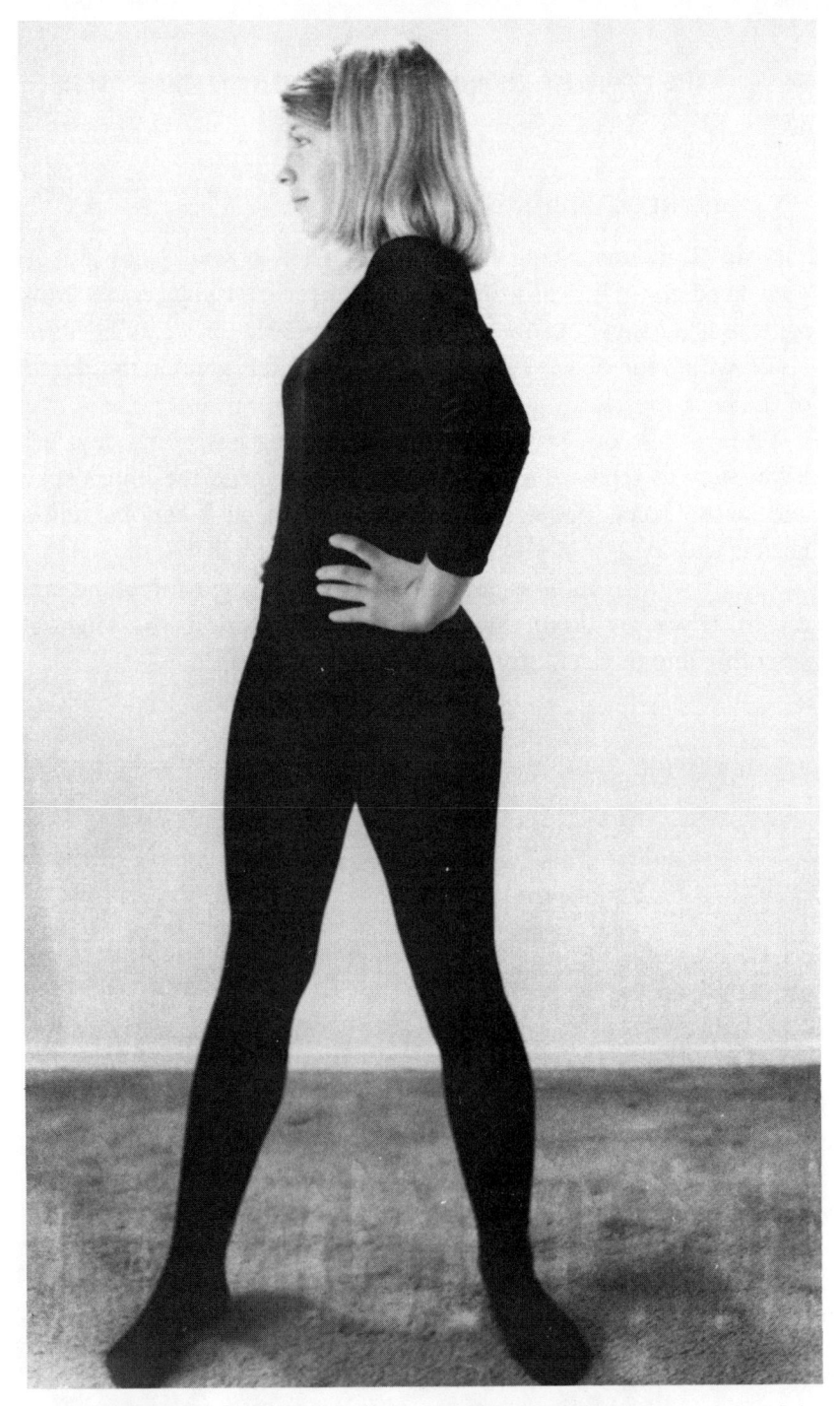

Twisting stretches the leg and lower trunk muscles as well as the muscles of the upper trunk. Try to avoid bending forward at the waist.

ARMS, NECK, AND SHOULDERS

Head Rotations. Stand relaxed with arms at your sides and let your head come forward until your chin rests on your chest. Now, roll the head slowly to the left and continue the roll making a full circle with your head. The wider the circle the greater the stretch of the neck muscles.

You can also do this sitting at a desk during a working day. It is a fine way to relieve the tension that builds up in the upper spine and neck. Some people have found that head rotations relieve headaches.

After several rotations in one direction, change directions and repeat. If you are doing this in the standing position, you might go smoothly into the trunk rotations described above.

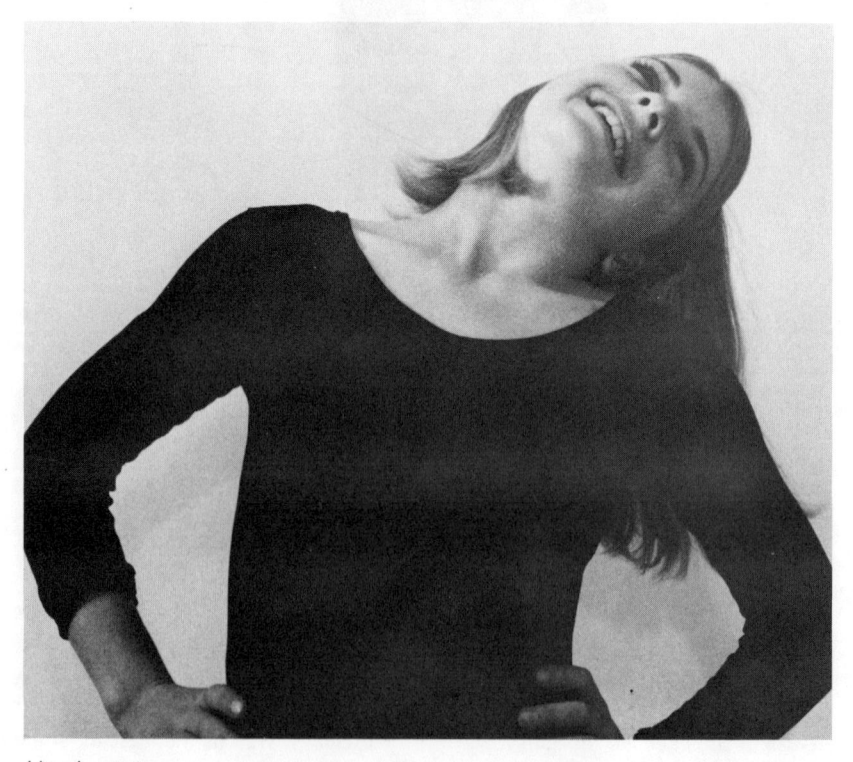

Head rotations.

PLIOMETRICS 57

Hand Waggles. Hold the arms up with elbows slightly bent and wrists relaxed. Now rotate your upper arms rapidly, making your hands waggle. Imagine that you are trying to shake water off your hands and fingers. This stretches upper arm muscles and does great

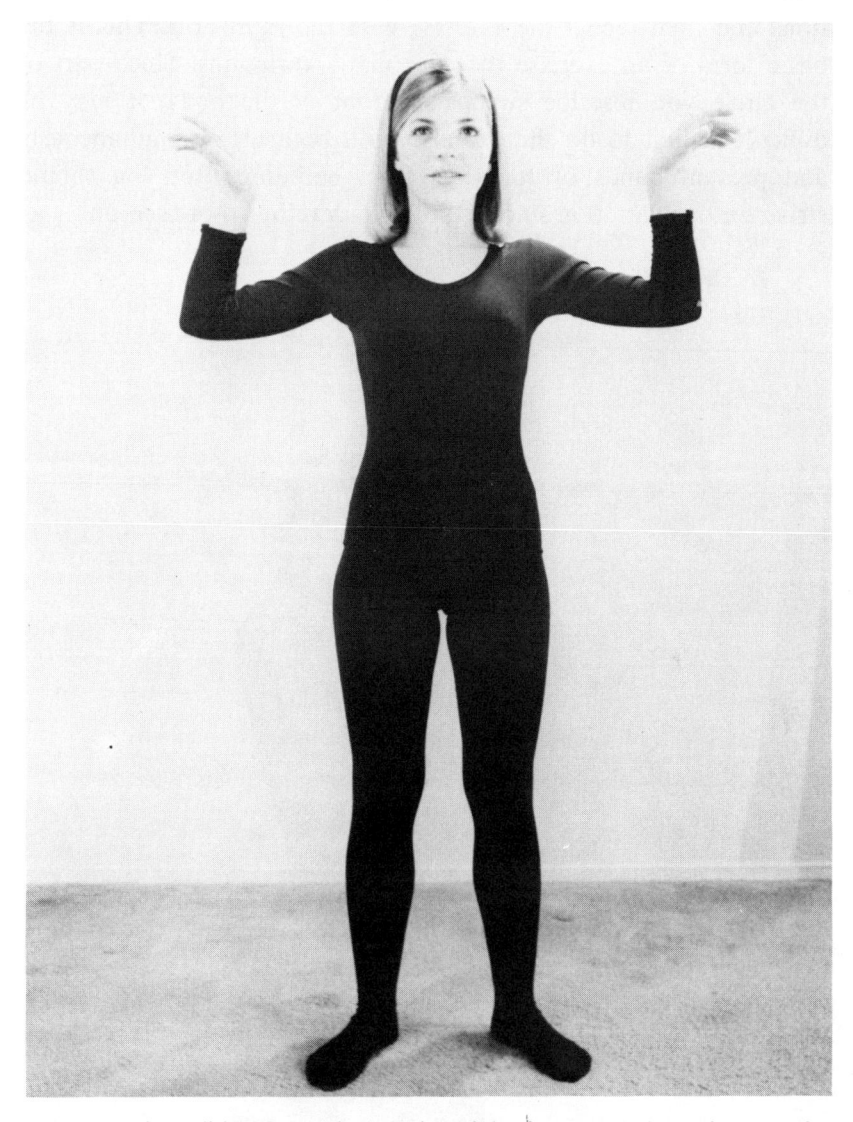

Hand waggles will loosen up the muscles of the forearm and stimulate circulation. You may want to do them while performing other exercises such as knee bends or stationary running.

things for circulation. If you can keep it up for half a minute your hands and arms will be tingling.

Arm Swings. With your right hand on your hip and your left arm hanging straight from the shoulder begin rotating the left arm so that your hand inscribes a big circle. Rotate the arm in both directions and then repeat the exercise with the right arm. This is the basic form of an exercise that has many variations. Since part of the circle you inscribe sweeps in front of the body, it may be difficult at first to do the exercise with both arms simultaneously and prevent hands or forearms from colliding. But you should strive for this variation since it will help develop co-ordination.

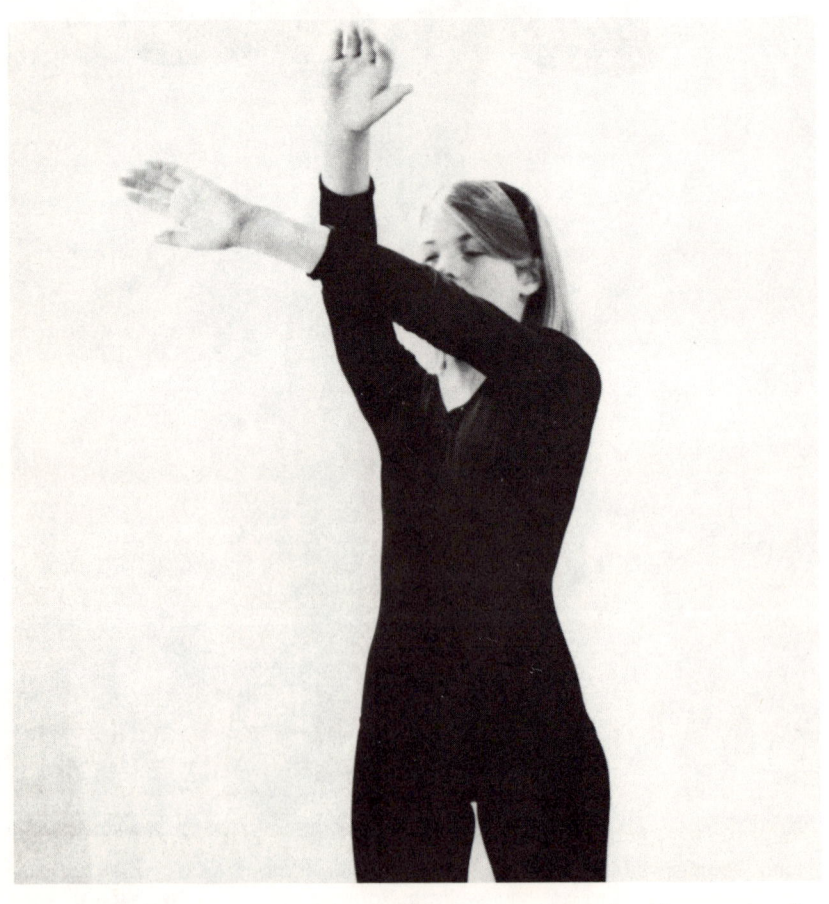

Arm swings stimulate circulation and loosen up arm and shoulder muscles. Begin swinging one arm at a time before you advance to the two-arm swing.

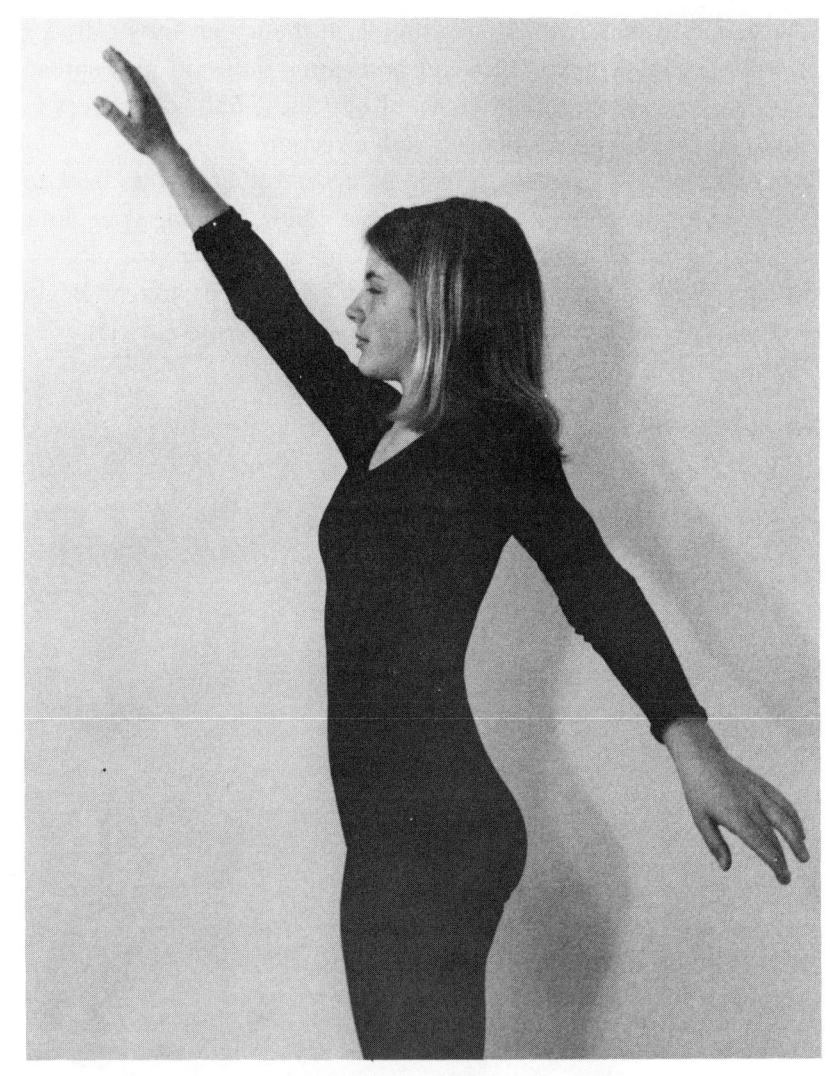

The crawl.

You might begin by doing the crawl, a variation of arm swings that will avoid collision. This copies the arm motion of the crawl stroke in swimming. As one arm is up, the other is down. Do the crawl with equal repetitions forward and backward. Try for full arm extension.

Arm swings limber the shoulder joints and muscles. They will also stimulate circulation.

60   THE COMPLETE BEGINNER'S GUIDE TO PHYSICAL FITNESS

A variation that concentrates stretch in the upper arms calls for inscribing smaller circles. Extend both arms sideways in a spread eagle position and inscribe circles of one-and-a-half to two feet in diameter. Do equal repetitions in both directions.

Pumps. Stand erect with your arms up and your elbows bent so that your forearms overlap at chest level. Now, keeping your arms at the same level, pump them back without unbending your elbows. Chest as well as shoulder muscles will get a good stretch. Begin slowly and avoid jerking motions that might pull tense muscles.

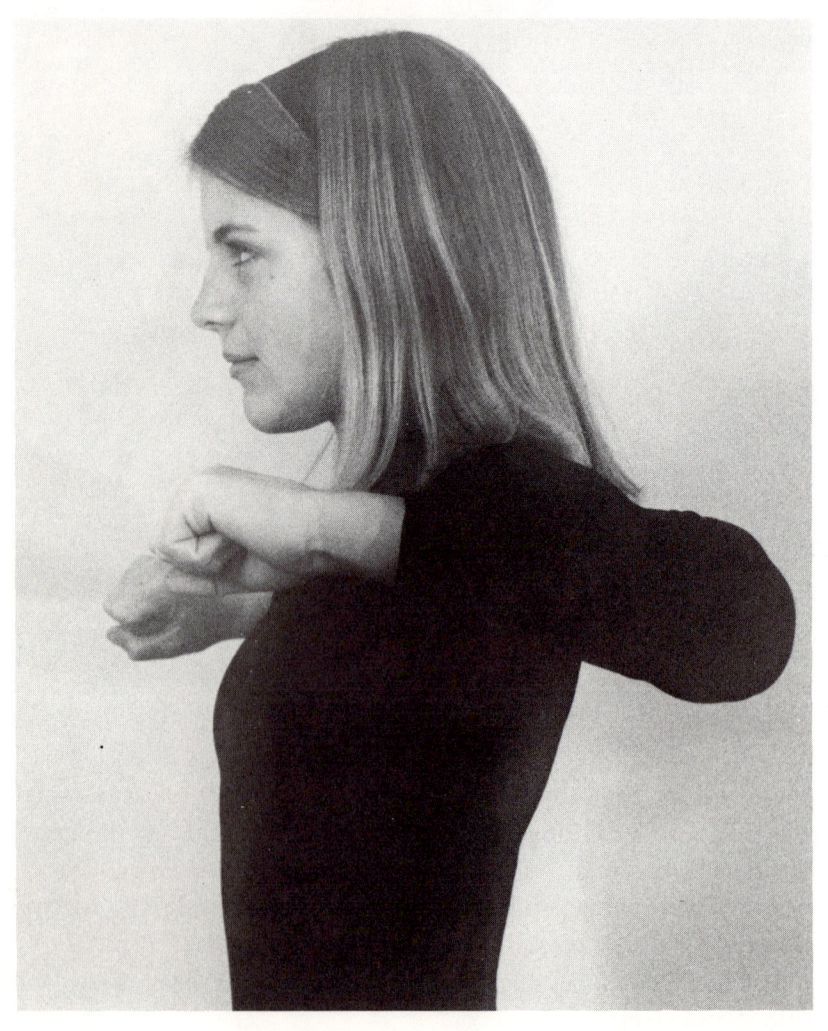

Elbow pumps.

PLIOMETRICS 61

LEGS

Bends. The standard bend has already been described in the first chapter. You should stick with this exercise until your legs are limber enough for you to touch the floor between your feet with no more than a slight bend of your knees. When you have reached this stage you can start exploring variations that will give greater

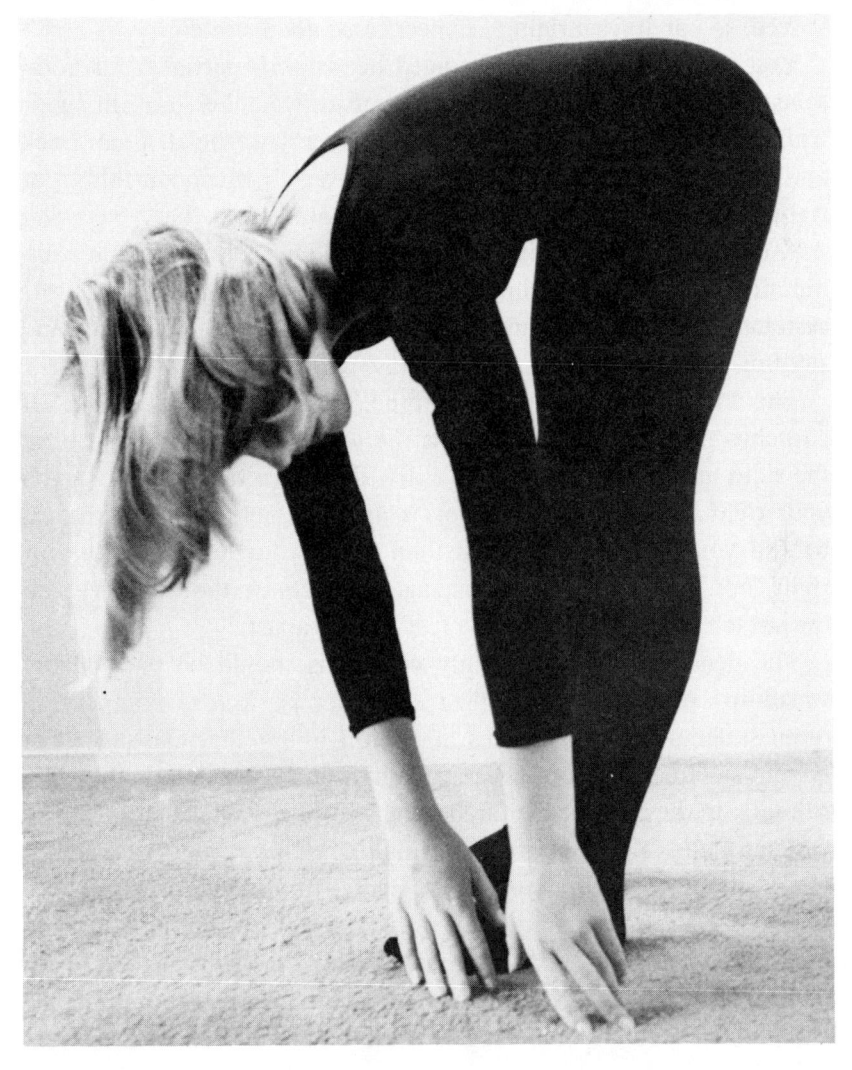

Advanced bend, touching outside feet.

stretch. First touch the fingertips of both hands to the floor on the outside of one foot and then the other. Return to the touch between the feet before you straighten up.

For more advanced work, touch outside and slightly behind each foot. Work at this until you can touch the knuckles of your closed fist to the floor. This often sounds impossible to beginners, but you will be reaching this stage sooner than you think. The muscles at the back of your legs which seem so tight now have a great deal of stretch in them. Some of the longest muscles of the body are involved, so you have a right to expect some good stretch.

You can combine your advanced bends with partial trunk rotations if you desire. After you touch outside your left foot, lift your trunk to the right with arms extended over your head. Lean back and then to the left before you bend over to touch outside your right foot. Now come up reversing the rotation so that you swing down to touch outside the left foot again. This is another fine combination exercise, stretching and flexing nearly all major muscle systems and giving the added bonus of increased circulation and rhythm.

The Pick. This is actually another variation on the bend. It stretches trunk muscles as well as the legs. Stand with arms out at the sides and feet about a yard apart. Bend over and turn to touch your right hand to your left foot. Your left arm should point aloft behind you. Straighten up and then touch your left hand to your right foot. Don't let your arms sag. To increase the difficulty and the stretch, do the pick with the feet farther apart.

The bend or one of its many variations should be part of any warm-up. Athletes who neglect this exercise before competition often suffer pulled hamstrings, a painful injury that can put them on the sidelines for weeks. The hamstring muscle is that big one running up the back of the thighs to the buttocks.

Knee Pulls. You can do these thigh stretchers either in a standing position or lying on your back. However, you will probably find it easier to keep your back straight if you are on the floor. Lifting one knee, grab your leg about midway down the shin and pull with both arms until the knee touches your chest. Keep the unused leg straight. You should feel a tug in the buttocks as well as the thigh.

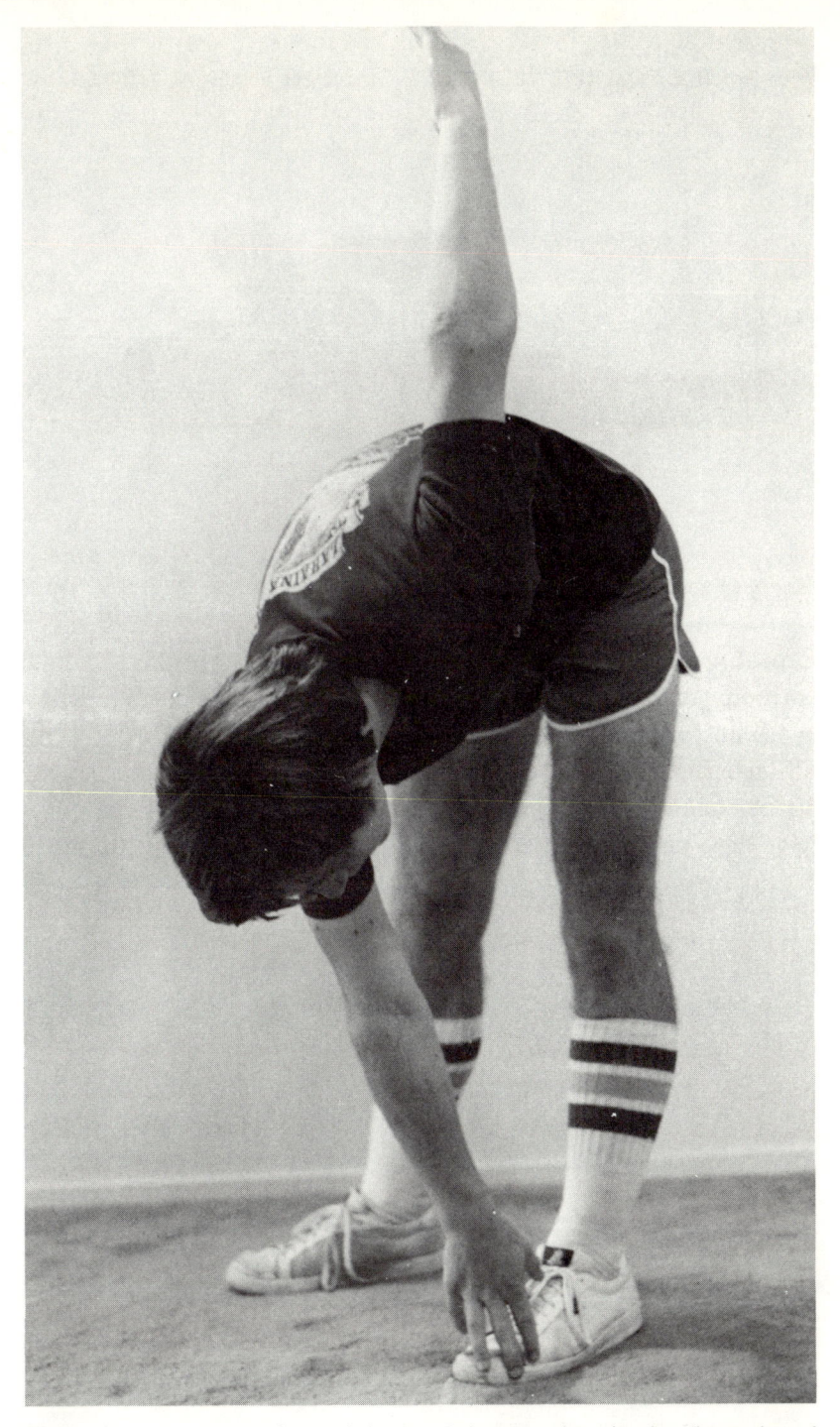

The pick is an advance form of the bend that stretches nearly all muscles of the body. The vigorous motion involved makes it a good cooling-off exercise.

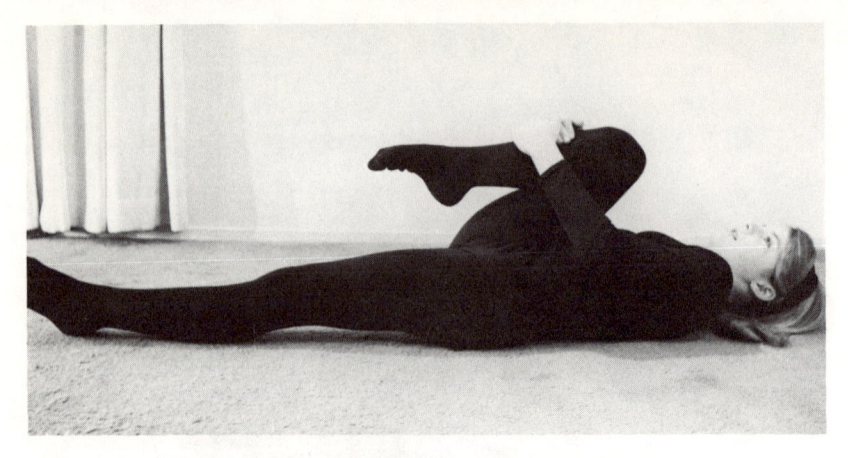

Knee pulls are best done as a floor exercise. The back and the extended leg must remain straight for maximum benefit.

Repeat with the other leg. If you do this exercise in the standing position, you can avoid bending the trunk forward to meet the knee by leaning against a wall.

Single Leg Lift. This combines stretching of the legs with flexing of the abdominal muscles. In the simplest form, leg lifts are done lying on your back with arms at your sides, lifting one leg at a time.

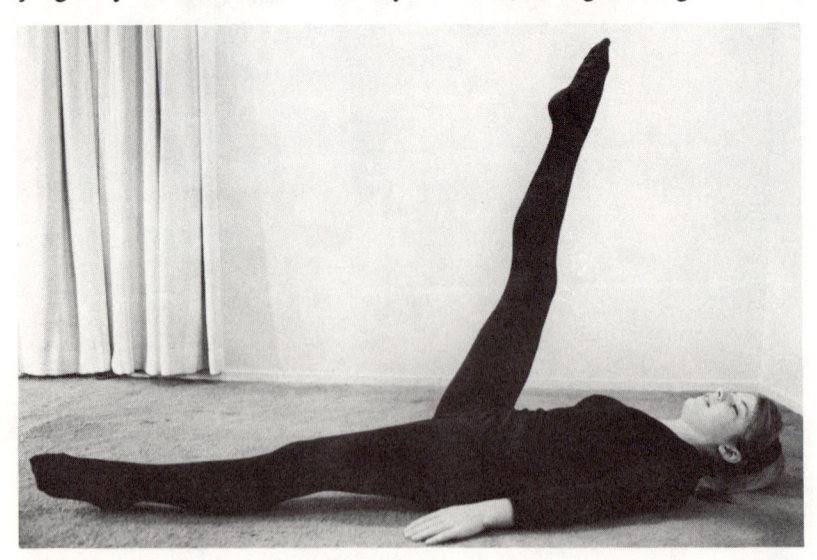

Single leg lifts flex the abdominal muscles while stretching the legs. Try for maximum lift of one leg while keeping the other extended.

PLIOMETRICS

Bring the leg as high as you can without bending the knee. The leg not in action should be flat on the floor. Repeat, alternately lifting one leg and then the other.

Double Leg Lifts. Lie on your back with your feet together and your arms at your sides. Lift both your legs as high as you can

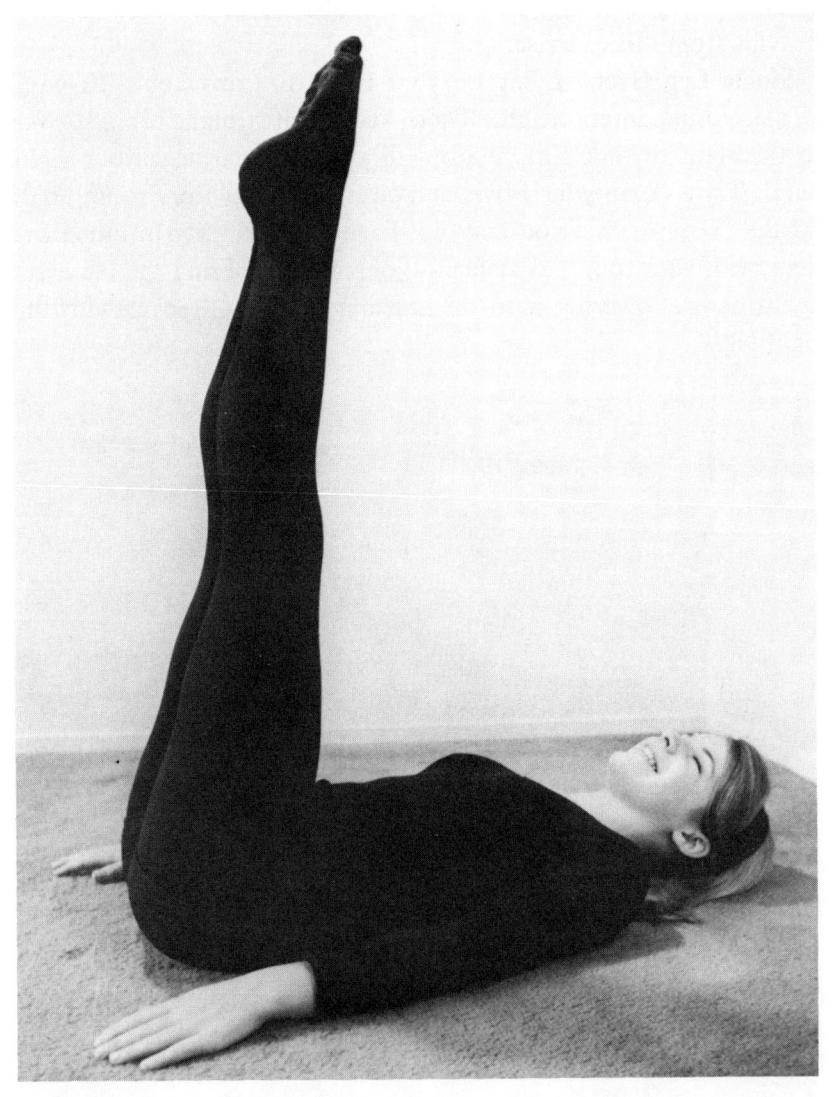

Double leg lifts combine stretching and flexing. From this position, you can lift your hips from the floor to add abdominal flex and give a stretch to the lower back.

without bending your knees. By bracing your arms on the floor, you will be able to lift your hips. Hold your maximum lift for a few seconds, trying not to let your legs sway. Now tuck your knees to your chest, lower your hips, extend your legs and return to the starting position.

You will get strong flex and a challenge in balance as side benefits from this exercise.

Single Leg Overs. Lying on your back with arms out, lift your left leg to maximum height. Then, keeping it straight bring it over to the right to touch the floor with your big toe near your right hand. Try to keep your pelvis and your shoulders from rolling half off the floor. At first you may not have the flexibility to touch the floor with your foot. Go as far as you can, then bring the leg erect again before lowering it to the starting position. Repeat with the right leg.

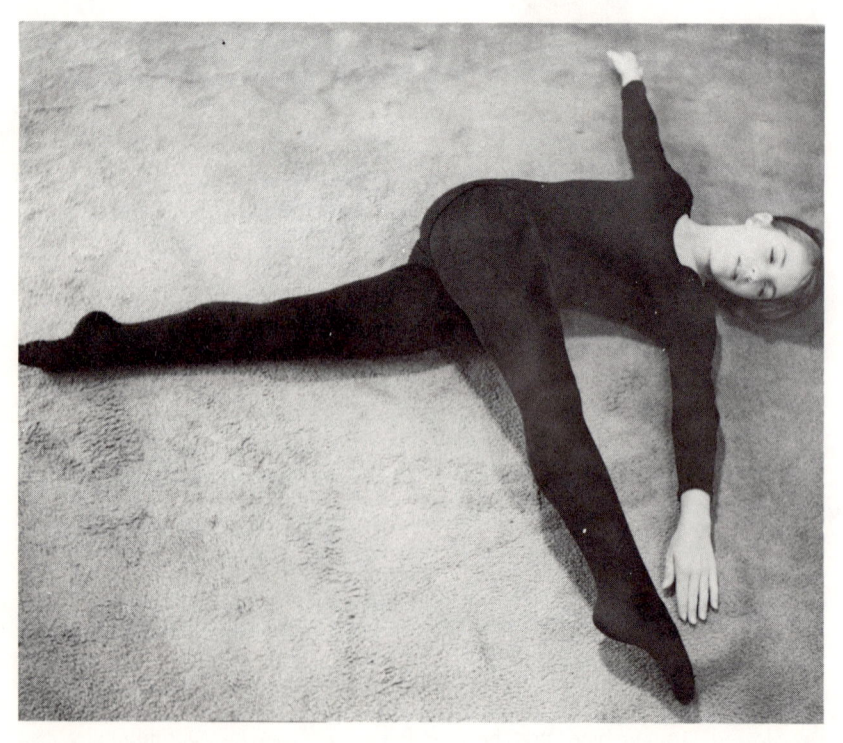

Single leg overs should be done without lifting the shoulders so that most of the flex is in the hips and lower back.

PLIOMETRICS

Double Leg Overs. Starting in the same position as above, bring both legs up together. Then swing them to the right, touching the feet to the floor close to your right hand. Lift them and swing to the left to touch. Now return to the starting position. Again, try not to let the pelvis roll. The legs should turn from the hip joints.

As a variation, do leg overs with the knees bent, trying to touch the floor with one knee and then the other, first to the right and then to the left.

Leg overs demand flexibility that usually does not come quickly. Don't be discouraged by your limitations. As long as you feel those leg muscles stretch, you are benefiting from these exercises.

Hurdler's Stretch. Take a hurdler's position on the floor with your left leg extended before you and your right leg at your side with your knee bent so that the foot points behind you. The farther back

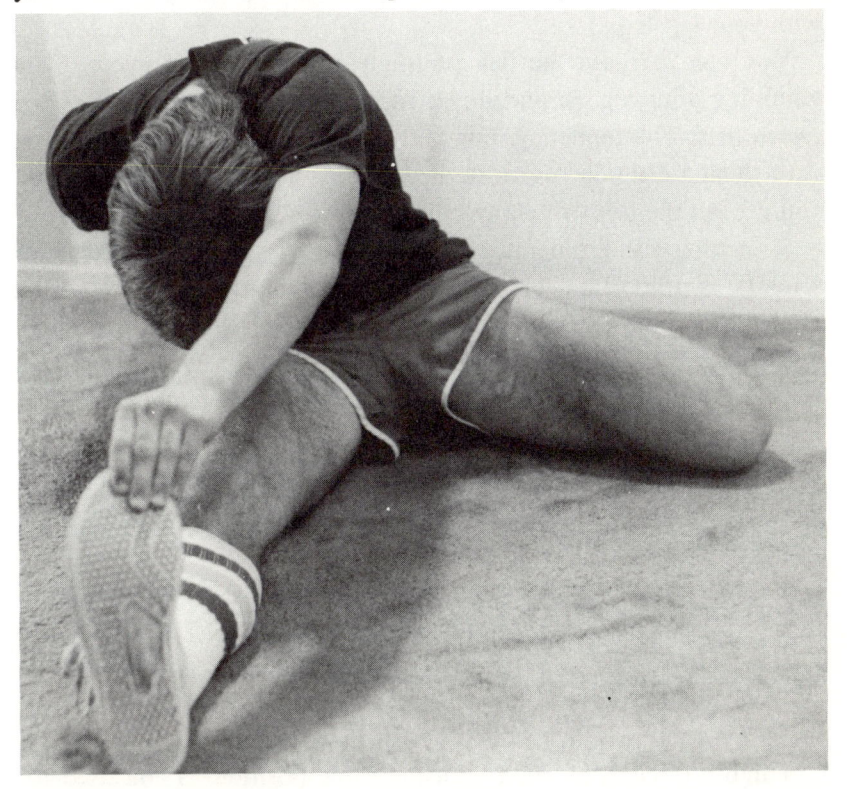

The hurdler's stretch, done as a warm-up exercise, is one of the best safeguards against groin pulls during sports. Twist your body to touch the foot with one hand and then the other. Then switch leg position.

you can get the bent leg, the more you will stretch the groin and thigh muscles. Now, with arms extended, turn and bend so you touch the toe of the front foot first with your left hand and then with your right. Count your touches and do the same number of repetitions with your right leg extended.

As a variation, you can simply bend forward, trying to touch your head to the knee of the extended leg. Hold the maximum forward position for a few seconds before repeating.

Scissors. Lie on your left side with your left arm stretched out on the floor above your head and your right hand braced on the floor in front of your chest. Raise your right leg, keeping it straight so it pivots upward from the hip joint. Get the best lift you can so that you get a strong tug in the groin. Lower the leg and repeat. Do several times and then reverse your position, repeating the exercise with your left leg.

You can increase the flex of thigh muscles in this exercise by whipping your leg up and down rapidly without letting it rest between lifts. The tendency, however, when doing this rapid motion, is to cheat a little on your lifts. If you don't swing that leg high, you will not get the full stretching benefit.

Stretching the groin muscle either with the hurdler's stretch or scissors is important before sports, particularly those requiring abrupt stop-and-go running such as basketball, baseball, football, and soccer. Pulled groin muscles, which can put you out of action for several days, are all too common in these sports and too often the injury is due to improper warm-up.

Back Kicks. Take the position of a sprinter at the starting line. The left leg should be extended and the right leg bent underneath your chest. Position your hands on the starting line and lift up on your toes. Now, rocking forward to put more weight on your hands, lift your feet and switch leg position with a rapid kick and tuck.

This exercise loosens leg muscles and also increases pulse and breathing rate. It is an excellent warm-up for jogging and running.

Thigh Stretcher. Starting with the same position as you used for back kicks, you can do a modified push-up that will put a strong stretch on the muscles at the front of the thigh. Position your feet a

PLIOMETRICS

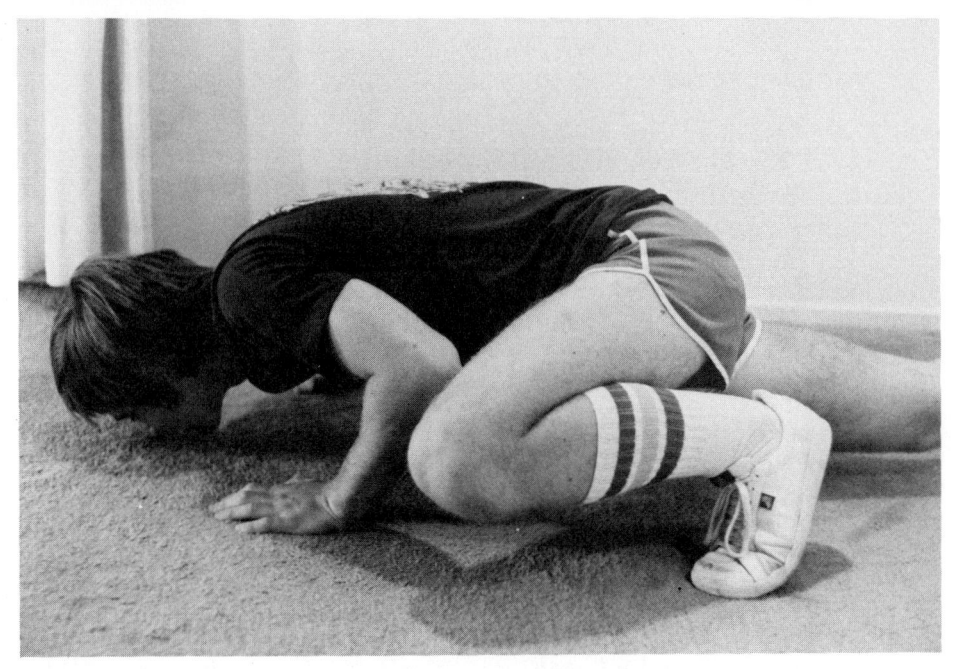

A good thigh stretching exercise is done from the starting position using back kicks. It also gives the arm and shoulder muscles the same flex they would get in a push-up.

little farther apart than you had them for the kicks. Now lower yourself to the floor until your hips touch. The bent leg should line up alongside the body. If you do not feel a tug in the thigh muscles, try shifting the leg back a few inches. Keep shifting until you find the position that makes this exercise work for you.

Jumping Jacks. Stand with your feet together and your arms at your side. Jump briskly, and while in the air, spread your feet and raise your arms. When you hit the floor, your feet should be about a yard apart and your arms should form a wide V above your head. Now jump again and come down in the starting position. Repeat rapidly.

This is a traditional exercise left over from the old calisthenic routines. It demands vigorous stretching and flexing, develops balance and co-ordination, and stimulates heart beat and breathing —in short, a great combination exercise.

6 *Miometrics*

Here you will be challenged by limits. Although the line between pliometics and miometrics is often not a sharp one, you will discover at once that exercises designed to flex certain sets of muscles have very definite limits, limits set by the present strength of these muscles.

You may have experienced little difficulty in repeating many of the pliometric exercises. Some of them actually get easier as muscle stretch increases during their performance. This will not be true with miometrics.

You may, for instance, be able to begin with just five sit-ups. That sixth sit-up will be impossible. Your muscles will simply refuse to do the job. This may be discouraging at first, particularly if you have a friend who can do twenty right off without batting an eye.

Don't lose heart. Your limits are not permanent. You will extend them rapidly with steady work. Perform up to your limit each day, and the day will soon come when you can do that sixth sit-up. Perhaps that will be your limit for the next several days, but then another breakthrough will come. In two months, the chances are good that you, too, will be doing twenty sit-ups. And you can bet that the achievement will give you great satisfaction.

MIOMETRICS

The guidelines for selecting miometric exercises for your program also differ. While you want to do enough stretching to involve all major muscle systems of the body, your flexing exercises should suit your individual needs.

The tests described in Chapter 4 will help point up these needs, but often performance of the exercises themselves will tell you clearly where more work is necessary.

If your performance of sit-ups is indeed poor, for instance, you must work at the exercise daily to extend your limit.

You must also consider all the other exercises in your program when selecting miometrics. Aerobic exercises usually give your legs plenty of flexing but, with the exception of swimming, they do not do much for the back, arm, shoulder, and abdominal muscles.

Some of the stretching exercises, as pointed out, require strong flexing. Here again, let this guide your selection of miometrics. For instance, if you are doing several leg lifts, particularly double leg lifts, your abdominal muscles are being flexed. In this case, there may be no need to make sit-ups a big part of your program.

Again, the exercises that follow are grouped by areas affected and are generally arranged in increasing order of difficulty.

ABDOMEN

Sit-ups. This exercise and its variations have already been covered in some detail in the first chapter, but this is a good place to stress the importance of strong abdominal muscles. These muscles are not only a major link between hips and trunk, but they also form a protective and supporting wall for the stomach, intestines, and other internal organs. When this wall becomes weak it sags into a pot belly. This is unattractive, but worse, it does not give those internal organs the support they need. The situation invites digestive disorders and problems with other internal functions.

Furthermore, that pot belly interferes with mobility. It simply gets in your way. That's all the more reason to be rid of it.

If sit-ups are impossible at first, start with head and shoulder curls. Lie on your back with your hands resting on your upper thighs. Curl forward, lifting your head and then your shoulders from the floor so that your fingers slide down your thighs almost to your knee caps. Do not lift the small of your back from the floor. Now uncurl slowly, letting your shoulders and then your head return to the floor.

Once you have mastered conventional sit-ups try to stick with a curling lift and descent. It is easier to do sit-ups with a stiff back, bending only at the hips, but you get more benefit from the curling motion.

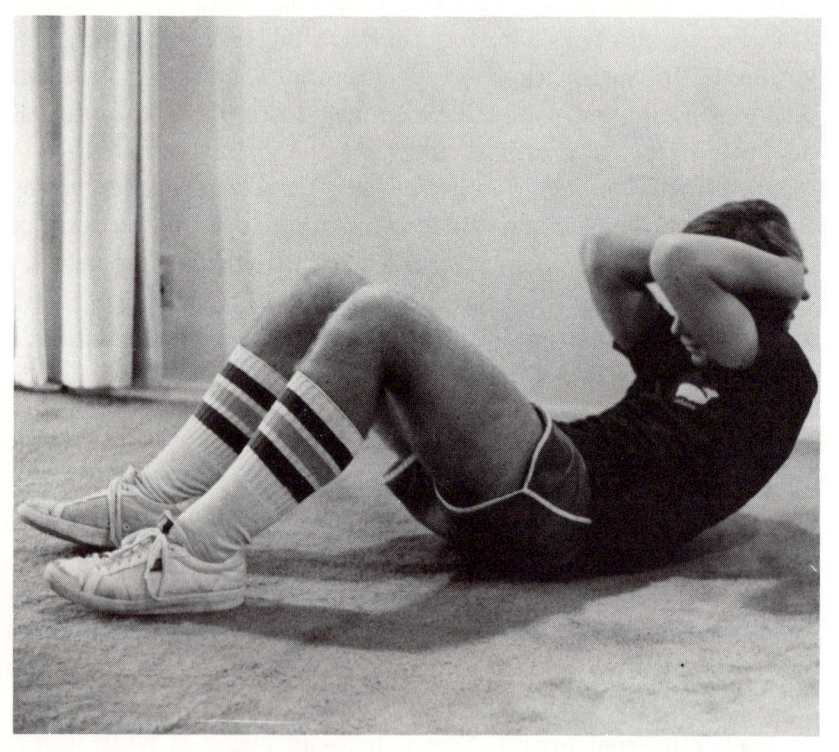

Sit-ups with the knees bent eliminate use of the psoas muscles and thus make the abdominals do all the work.

You will increase the benefit even more when you can do sit-ups with your knees bent and your feet flat on the floor. This position eliminates use of the long psoas muscles which run through the pelvis, connecting the thighs with the lower back. Sitting up with bent knees makes the abdominals do all the work.

Twisting Sit-ups. Sitting up with your hands clasped behind your neck and touching an elbow to the opposite knee has already been described. To get more twist, lie on your back with your feet about twenty inches apart and your arms at your sides. Now sit up and try to touch a hand to the opposite foot. This variation will give the muscles of the buttocks and the back of the legs a good stretch. Swing to touch the other foot with the other hand before you return to the starting position.

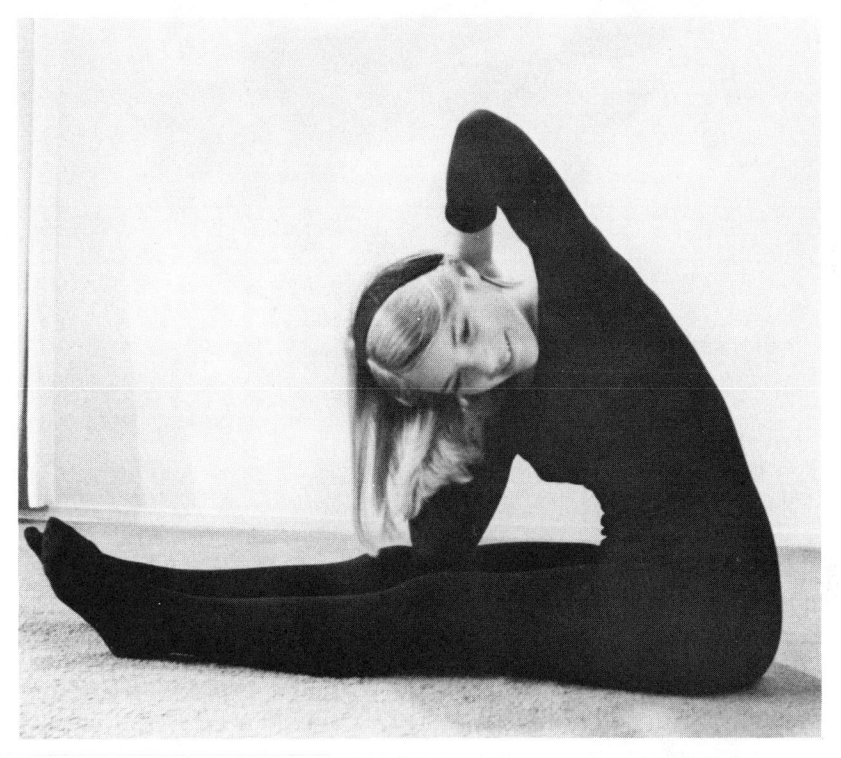

Twisting sit-up, touching elbow to opposite knee.

Rocking V's. Lie on your back with hands about six inches from your sides and feet about two feet apart. Curl up to a sitting position so that your trunk is at a ninety-degree angle with your legs. Hold that angle as you lean back, letting your legs rise. Stop when trunk and legs are at a forty-five-degree angle with the floor. Next rock forward returning your legs to the floor. Then lean back

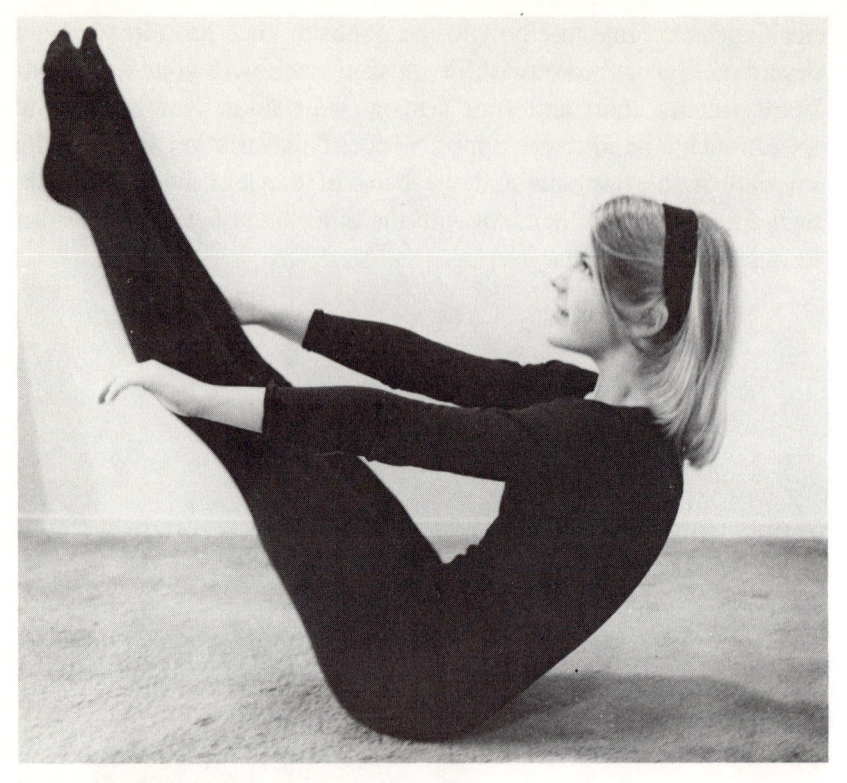

Rocking V's, another advanced sit-up exercise, are a good test of balance as well as a good way to flex the abdominals.

slowly to the starting position. This not only strengthens abdomen, thighs, and back but also helps develop balance and agility. Rocking V's probably will not be easy for you, but in case you want to add difficulty, try the exercise without going to the sitting position. In other words, lift both legs and trunk simultaneously so that they are at a forty-five-degree angle with the floor. Hold this balanced V for a few seconds before easing trunk and legs back to the floor.

BACK

Leg Raises. Lie on your stomach. Rest your chin on a hand and bring your feet close together. Without bending your knees, raise one leg and then the other as high as possible from the floor. Point your toes for full extension. This exercise is one of several that will strengthen the large flat muscle covering the lower back. Weakness of this muscle, the erector spinae, is a common cause of backache. The erector and many other muscles surrounding it support the spine like guy wires on a mast.

Leg Whips. Starting from the same position, lift both feet about two inches from the floor. Now, without bending the knees, lift one foot and then the other in rapid whipping motion without letting your feet touch the floor. When you can do leg whips in this manner for at least thirty seconds without pause, you should advance to the raised trunk position. Start with your hands at your sides, palms up, and your chin on the floor. Now do your leg whips with your shoulders and chest as far off the floor as possible. Your weight should rest on your hips and your hands. How high you lift your feet with each whip is not as important as the effort you put into the exercise.

Leg and Trunk Lifts. Lie on your stomach with your feet together and your hands clasped in the small of your back. Without bending your knees, lift your legs and your trunk. At the same time, straighten your arms and stretch them back, forcing your

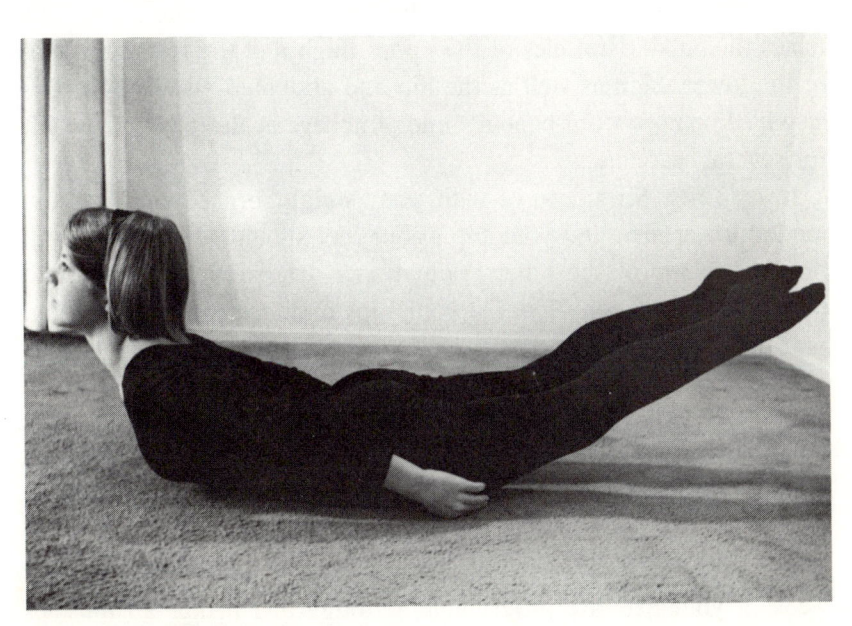

Leg and trunk lifts strengthen the muscles of the lower back. Your weight eventually should rest on your hips alone when you reach maximum lift.

clasped hands toward your heels. Return slowly to the starting position and repeat. The arm lift in this exercise should force your shoulder blades together and flex muscle along your entire back. These lifts are often recommended to correct poor posture.

Spreads and Flutters. Both these exercises begin from the same position. Lie on your stomach with arms and legs extended. For the spread, lift trunk and legs and simultaneously swing your arms and legs wide. Bring them together again and return to the starting position. For the flutter, lift your trunk and legs and whip arms and legs up and down without touching the floor. The left arm goes up as the right leg rises. The right arm goes up with the left leg. Spreads and flutters are about as close as you can come to swimming motions without getting wet. They bring many muscles into play and limber both shoulder and hip joints.

LATERAL MUSCLES

Two-leg Lift. Lie on one side with your lower arm outstretched to cushion your head. Brace the palm of your other hand on the floor in front of your chest. Now, lift both legs from the floor. This flexes the outside muscles of the upper thigh and the inside muscles of the lower thigh as well as the hip and abdomen muscles. Do this slowly. For maximum benefit, hold your legs at the peak of the lift for several seconds.

Body Lifts. Sit sideways with your weight braced on your extended lower arm and your hip. Your feet should be together with one leg on top of the other. Your upper arm should be extended, parallel to your legs. Now lift your hips and straighten your body, putting all your weight on your lower arm and your feet as you lift your upper arm above your head. Hold for a few seconds before lowering slowly to the starting position. Hips and thighs and the muscles of the entire trunk should get a good flex from this exercise. It is also good balance training. If balance is a problem at first, brace your feet against a wall.

Leg Extensions. Don't expect to master this exercise in the first week of your exercise program. It is tough and brings all muscles from the shoulders to the tip of your toes into play. Do the body lift

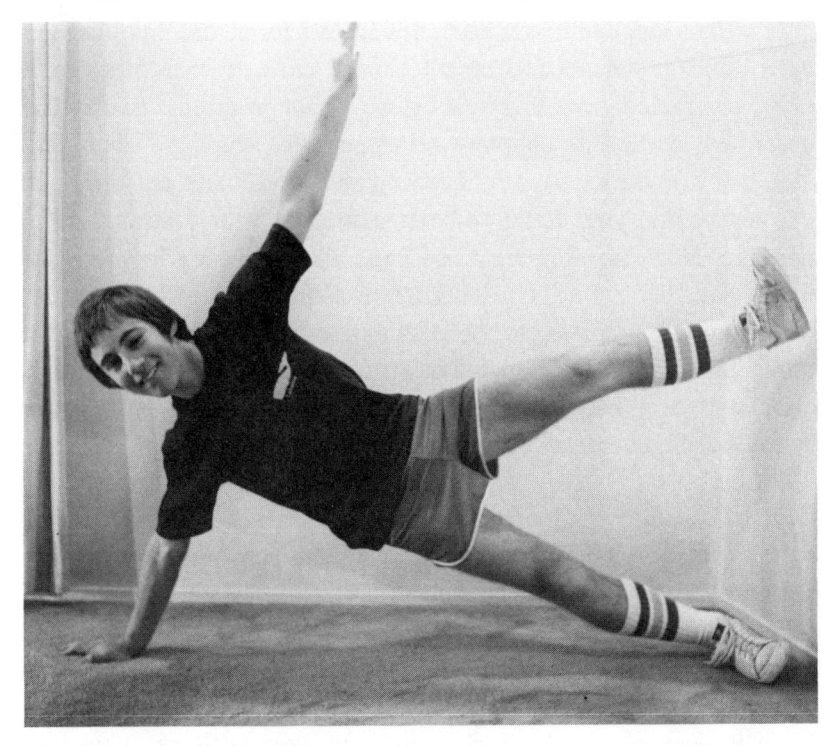

Leg extensions are tough. Don't expect to do as many repetitions of this exercise until your lateral muscles are well developed.

with your upper hand clasped behind your neck. Now lift your upper leg sideways as high as possible. Lower it slowly to the lower leg and repeat. Again, if balance is a problem, use a wall as a foot brace.

The chances are that lateral exercises will introduce you to muscles you didn't know you had. The exercises are especially useful for weight watchers who tend to put fat on hips and thighs.

CHEST AND ARMS

Push-up Training. It's possible to make a strong argument against standard push-ups. They discourage people and turn them away from fitness programs probably more than any other single exercise. They are difficult. And, yes, they are important, but they are not important enough to kill your enthusiasm for all exercise.

If at first you cannot do push-ups in any form, don't be discouraged. You are in good company. Work hard at your other exercises, but include one that will train you for push-ups. Back kicks described in the last chapter will strengthen arms and shoulders. You can also do leg swings. Take a hands and knees position. Lift one leg behind you. Bend your knee to raise your foot as high as possible. Now, keeping the knee bent, swing the leg forward and under your body, bringing the knee as close to your chin as possible. Then return the leg to the starting position and repeat with the other leg. While this takes balance and gives your legs and hips a good stretch, it also shifts your weight forward, strengthening your arms and shoulders.

Pushing away from a wall also provides good push-up training. Try to keep your body straight, and stand far enough from the wall so that it takes real effort to push away. As you progress, position your feet a few inches farther from the wall. Eventually, you will be ready for push-ups.

Knee push-ups and standard push-ups have already been described. Don't think that you must advance beyond knee push-ups. If they demand good effort each time you perform them, the chances are that you will benefit more by repeating this exercise twenty times than you will struggling to do five standard push-ups.

Again, this comes down to an individual judgment that you must make yourself. As a general rule, however, most males should advance to standard push-ups and make them a regular part of their workouts. Well-muscled females should also advance, but females with naturally spare muscles should be content with knee push-ups.

Elbow Push-ups. If you have difficulty making the transition from knee to standard push-ups, try this exercise for a few weeks. Lie on your stomach with your feet together, your toes resting on the floor. Prop your shoulders and chest up with your elbows. Your forearms should be on the floor, pointing forward. Now straighten your body, lifting it entirely off the floor so that your weight is on your feet and your forearms. Ease your hips back to the floor and repeat. This will provide the extra strength in legs, back, and shoulders necessary for standard push-ups.

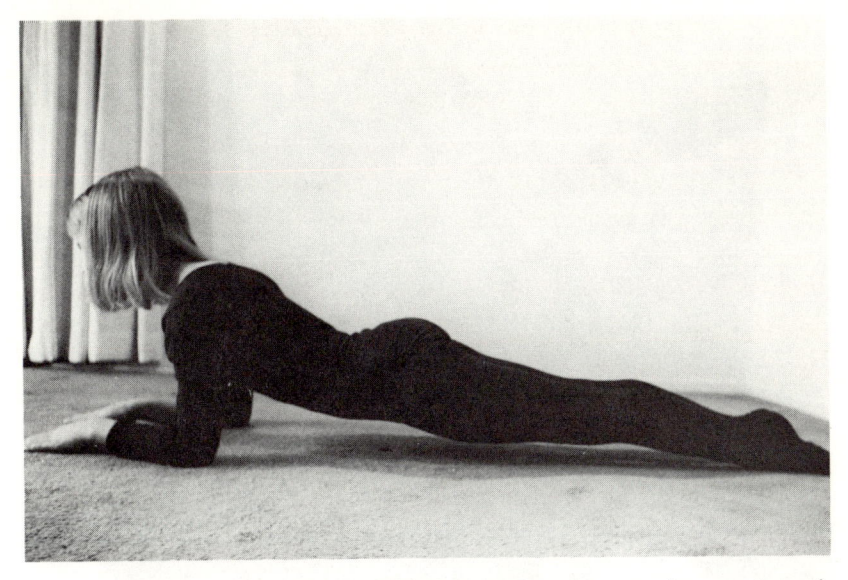

Elbow push-ups provide a good intermediate exercise between knee and standard push-ups.

Advanced Push-ups. Eventually, standard push-ups may become too easy for you. Body arches will make them more challenging. After you have touched your chin to the floor, arch your body from the waist to touch your forehead to the floor in back of your hands. Then straighten your arms and repeat, touching chin and forehead with your elbows bent.

Those who are athletic and well co-ordinated can find even more challenge by pushing up hard enough to lift their hands and either clap them together or slap them against the chest. You must move your hands quickly, getting them back on the floor before your body descends. The exercise requires explosive flexing of the arm and shoulder muscles and should not be attempted until you are in peak condition.

Pull-ups. This is the only miometric exercise listed here that requires special equipment, a parallel bar. Actually, an overhanging tree limb in your back yard or along the route of a customary walk can serve very well as a substitute. If you cannot find a co-operative tree, you can install a bar in a door frame, using a pipe with stout brackets.

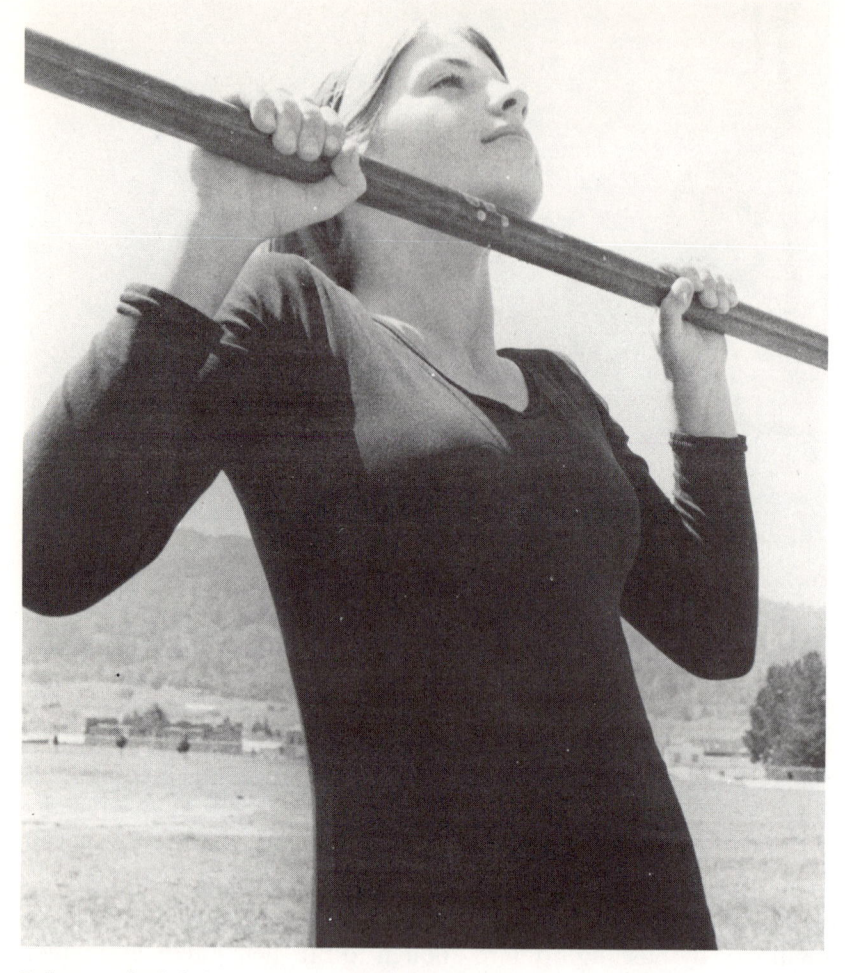

Pull-up on high bar.

The exercise, as already described in the Youth Fitness Test, can be done either with a low bar at chin level, or a high bar that will lift your feet off the floor when you grip it. In both cases, start with an overhand grip on the bar.

For the low bar exercise, place your feet slightly ahead of a vertical line from the bar. Keep your legs together and your body straight as you straighten your arms and lean away from the bar. Pull yourself up to chin the bar, keeping your elbows close to your body. Repeat as often as you can without strain.

MIOMETRICS

For tougher work on the high bar use the same straight-body form, tucking the elbows close to your sides. Do not kick your legs or let your body sway. Make your arms and shoulders do the work. Reversing the grip for pull-ups will bring a different set of forearm muscles into play, but the underhand grip tends to pull you into the bar. Be alert for this, or you may bump your nose.

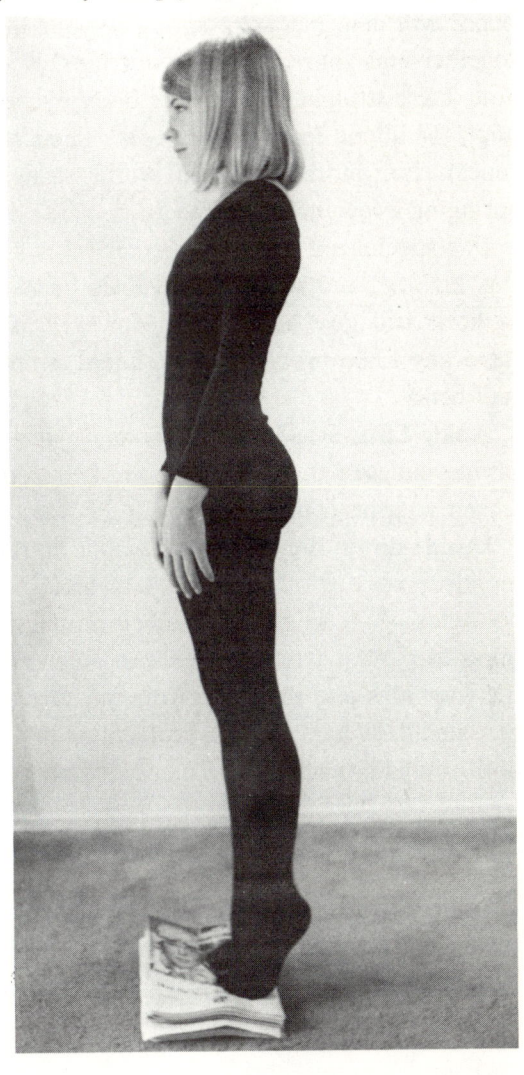

Ankle lifts may solve the sore ankle problems that might arise during the first few days of jogging or running. A wooden plank will give a firmer base than a stack of magazines.

LEGS

Knee Bends. Although your legs may get a full workout in the aerobic phase of your program, you may find when you begin jogging, jumping rope, or cycling that your legs tire quickly. Half knee bends will help put extra spring in your legs. Stand with your feet together and your hands on your hips. Keeping your head up and your back straight, lower your body by bending your knees to an angle of about forty-five degrees. Then straighten your legs and repeat. For more advanced work, straighten your legs rapidly, springing a few inches off the floor.

For specialized work, particularly for sports that require jumping, kicking, and sprinting full knee bends that bring the buttocks to heels will give added flex. However, if you are overweight or have any knee problems you should avoid full bends. Stick with half bends.

Ankle Lifts. Stand with the balls of your feet on a plank or stack of magazines so that your heels are two to three inches off the floor. Lower your heels until they touch the floor, then lift to your toes.

Upside-down Bicycles. This classic introduced in Chapter 1 as an ideal cooling-off exercise has many other benefits including good flex of the thigh and buttock muscles. It is excellent for trimming excess fat from these areas. Remember the higher you can lift your legs and the faster you can turn the "pedals" the greater the benefit. If balance is a problem at first, move your legs slowly until you gain confidence. Then speed up.

7   Aerobics

Thanks to Dr. Kenneth H. Cooper and his fitness program for the U. S. Air Force we can rate and compare the aerobic exercises in terms of training effect.

We can say, for instance, than ten minutes of skipping rope will produce the same training effect as twenty minutes of brisk walking, or that swimming 250 yards in five minutes is the equivalent of running a mile in twelve minutes and forty-five seconds.

What exactly is training effect? In very simple terms, it is the ability of your body to take in, absorb, and distribute oxygen. This, as we have seen, involves several body systems. A high rate of oxygen intake requires healthy lungs and strong muscles of the chest cavity. It requires a strong and efficient heart. It requires well-toned muscles throughout the body. And it requires a good circulatory system, with resilient blood vessels, free of obstruction and restrictions.

You can get a fair idea of the training effect an exercise produces by taking your pulse before and after a workout. Dr. Cooper, however, based his ratings on actual oxygen consumption measured with laboratory equipment. His primary standard was the amount of oxygen (measured in millimeters) processed in relation to the body weight of the subject (measured in kilograms) in one minute.

He found that degree of effort produced surprising variations. When a man on a treadmill jogged the equivalent of a mile in fourteen-and-a-half minutes, he processed seven millimeters of oxygen per kilogram of body weight per minute. When the man ran a mile in six-and-a-half minutes, however, the reading jumped to forty-two millimeters.

Different exercises at various performance rates produced further far-ranging readings, and to simplify the results, Dr. Cooper translated oxygen consumption rates to points.

This made possible an easy evaluation of many different exercises at a variety of different performance rates. The next step was to determine just how much exercise an individual must have to put all the oxygen processing systems in top condition.

After testing thousands of individuals and rating their fitness from poor to excellent, Dr. Cooper found that those in the excellent category were already exercising regularly. Using his point system to rate their exercises, he found that these people were "earning" thirty or more points a week.

This became the goal for his program. It is a goal suited for almost everyone. Generally, women must take longer in working up to the goal than men. Everyone over thirty should also pace themselves to avoid strain. But all, no matter what age or sex, should eventually have a thirty-point aerobic program.

Dr. Cooper has one reservation. He does not recommend heavy aerobic workouts for youngsters under eleven years old. On the other hand, he believes that thirty points may be too low for most teen-agers.

On first look at the point system this may seem to be a lot of exercise, but you may be earning many points right now without knowing it. If you participate in sports, if you walk or ride a bike to and from work or school, and if your work itself requires physical activity, you may already be close to a thirty-point goal.

The description of various aerobic exercises that follow will help you rate your current activities as well as plan a program.

STATIONARY RUNNING

You have already learned how to do this exercise, and you know how to check your pulse rate to make sure you put the necessary effort into your performance. According to Dr. Cooper, five minutes of running at a rate of seventy to eighty steps a minute is worth one-and-a-half points. Ten minutes is worth three points. Twenty minutes will give you six points.

To earn thirty points a week, you must do twenty minutes of stationary running five days a week, or a total of an hour and forty minutes a week. It is possible, however to cut down on the time by increasing your effort. If you can lift your pace to eighty to ninety steps a minute and lift your feet eight inches instead of four inches from the floor with each step, you will earn two points in five minutes, four points in ten minutes, and six points in fifteen minutes. Five fifteen-minute sessions a week, a total of an hour and fifteen minutes, will earn thirty points.

Though it may not be the most exciting way to earn points, stationary running does have some solid advantages over other exercises. You need no special clothing. Pajamas or underwear will serve nicely. And you can workout in bare feet to enjoy an unshod freedom that has become all too rare. An exception in this relaxed dress code must be made, however, for girls with large breasts who should wear a good, supportive bra for any jogging, running, or jumping exercise.

Of course, as an indoor exercise, stationary running can be done in any weather. Also, with no one staring at you, you need not feel self-conscious. This seems to be particularly important for beginners, many of whom are unduly embarrassed to be seen jogging down a sidewalk.

As with any exercise you must set your own rate of progress. In the beginning, two minutes of stationary running may be your limit. Work to that limit every day for a week. Then begin adding to it.

In actual practice, the limits in aerobics rise abruptly. You may have to struggle to reach four minutes a day, but then suddenly, you will be able to run in place for ten minutes without strain or fatigue.

SKIPPING ROPE

Another exercise you can perform indoors, skipping rope contributes to co-ordination, agility, and balance while producing an aerobic training effect. In Dr. Cooper's ratings, skipping rope is on a par with stationary running. Ten minutes of skipping is worth three points.

There are, however, some advantages over stationary running. For one thing, the rope forces you into a rhythm that will not allow your effort to dwindle. This is all too easy with stationary running where you must make a conscious effort to bring your feet high and maintain a steady pace.

Skipping rope, once you have mastered it, becomes almost mechanical. If you have never jumped rope, it's time you learned.

Take a length of Number 10 sash cord or the equivalent. You can buy a fancy rope with swivel handles later if you wish, but a plain cord is all you need at the beginning. Find your length by standing on the middle of the cord and bring the ends up under your arms. Tie overhand knots at the points where the rope is even with your armpits.

Now you have your rope, but it is a good idea to do your first practice jumps without it. Stand with your feet together, your elbows in, and your hands about a foot out from your hips. Now start bouncing on the balls of your feet. Do this briskly, trying for a rate of seventy to eighty bounces a minute.

You may not be able to keep this up for a full minute at first. Bounce for half a minute, rest, and bounce for half a minute again. Once you have established a steady rhythm, stop and practice rope swinging.

Take both ends of the rope in one hand and swing it so that the looped end just grazes the floor. This doesn't take a great deal of hand motion. Practice until you can swing the rope smoothly with

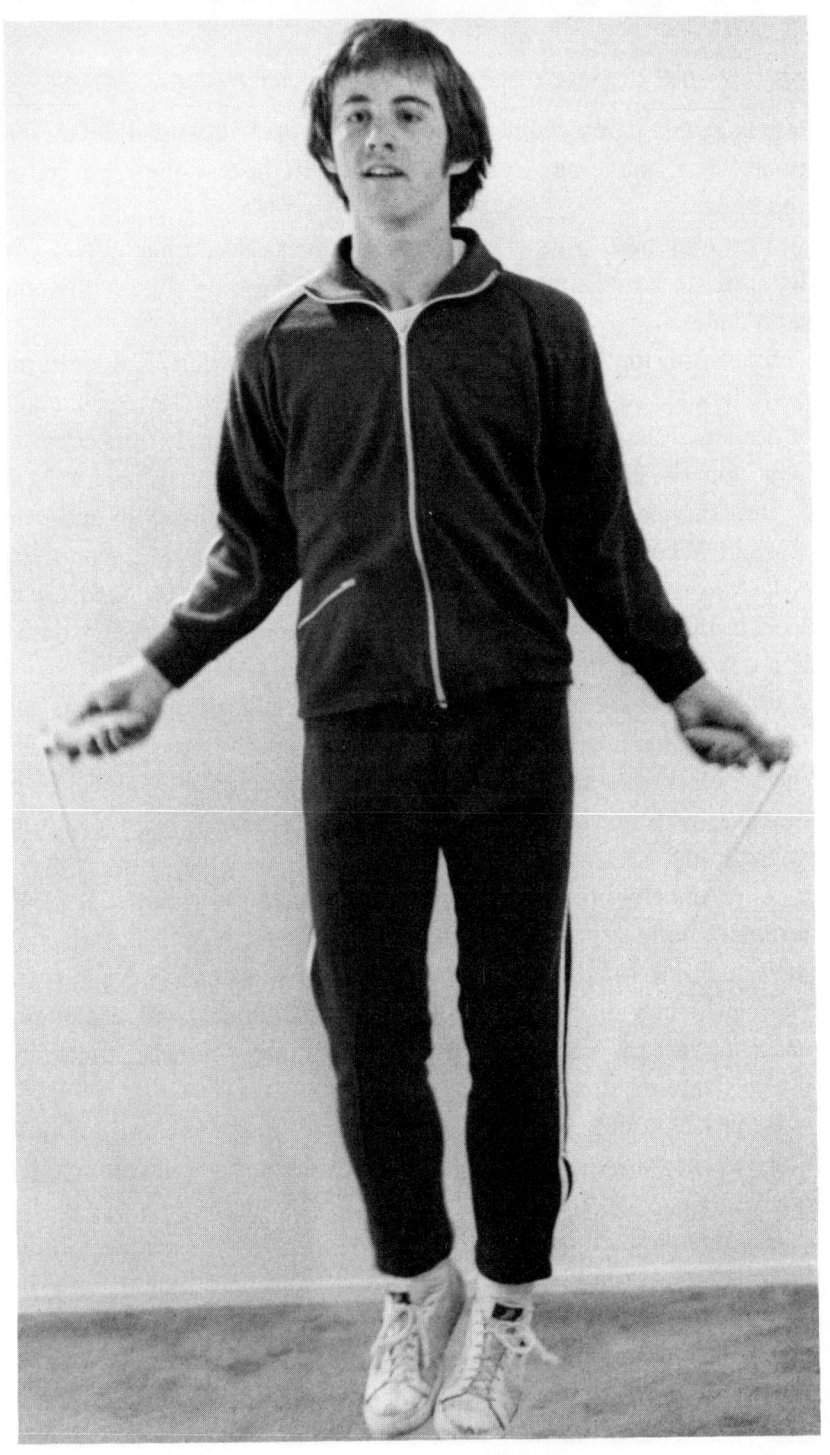

Skipping rope takes some skill to master, but it is worth the effort. The rope forces you to hold a good rhythm with no letup during your workout.

either hand. Then, while swinging the rope at your side in one hand, start bouncing, so that your feet lift just as the rope grazes the floor.

You may need several sessions to perfect this timing. When you have mastered it, however, you can begin skipping rope with some confidence.

Start with the loop behind you. Bring it over your head and time your bounce to let the rope pass under your feet. You will make mistakes at first, but stick with it. When timing and form come to you, you will be off like a rabbit.

Best skipping form calls for an erect body with head up and eyes straight ahead. Watching the rope or looking down at your feet will destroy your timing. Land on the balls of your feet and try to land in the same spot with each bounce. Most of the spring should come from your ankles, not your knees.

Once you have mastered this simple or plain bounce, you can advance to the rhythm bounce. This calls for an extra bounce when the rope is in the air. It takes more effort, but you may make fewer mistakes with this advanced step. That extra bounce helps you hold your timing.

After the rhythm bounce, you can move to the running step, alternately bouncing on one foot and then the other. This step may have a cosmetic advantage over the first two steps. There is some good evidence that the plain and rhythm bounce will eventually cause large calf muscles. If this is something you wish to avoid, use the running step.

Peter L. Skolnik in his book *Jump Rope!* recommends maximum daily workouts of fifteen minutes for women and seventeen minutes for men.

Beginners must build gradually. In the first week, females should jump no more than two minutes a day and males should jump no more than three minutes a day. Skolnik says those under thirty years old can build to their maximums in ten weeks. Those thirty to thirty-nine should use a twelve-week program. Those forty to forty-nine should take fourteen weeks, and those over fifty should take sixteen weeks to reach their maximums.

WALKING

Pace again determines the training effect. If you stroll along, taking twenty minutes or more to cover a mile, you will earn no aerobic points. Brisk walking, however, is one of life's best exercises, and it's also fine recreation.

Walking at a five-mile-an-hour clip is worth two points for each mile. Walking at a four-mile-an-hour clip is worth one point a mile. If you walked a little more than two fast miles every day of the week, you would earn your thirty points. You could do this by spending no more than twenty-six minutes a day on a favorite walk.

When you walk, let your arms swing freely and make a conscious effort to extend your stride. Don't expect to start right out at top speed. Begin slowly. Amble part of the way if you start getting winded. Stop and rest if you feel tired.

If you plan to make walking your main aerobic exercise, select a route you can measure with your car's odometer. Several routes, if they are available, will give you day-to-day variety.

Walk at least two miles every day. It may take you an hour when you begin, but as your condition improves, you will be able to increase your pace week by week.

If your schedule does not allow you time for this kind of program, you can at least try to fit walking in as part of your daily routine. Get off your bus a few blocks from work and walk the rest of the way. If you need something at the corner store, leave the car in the garage and do the errand on foot.

You need no special outfit. Comfortable clothing and sturdy, well-fitted shoes are the only requirements for walking.

JOGGING AND RUNNING

Jogging pace can vary all the way from four miles an hour—a good walking pace—up to seven miles an hour. Anything faster than that is running.

Again, the faster you go, the greater the training effect. Under

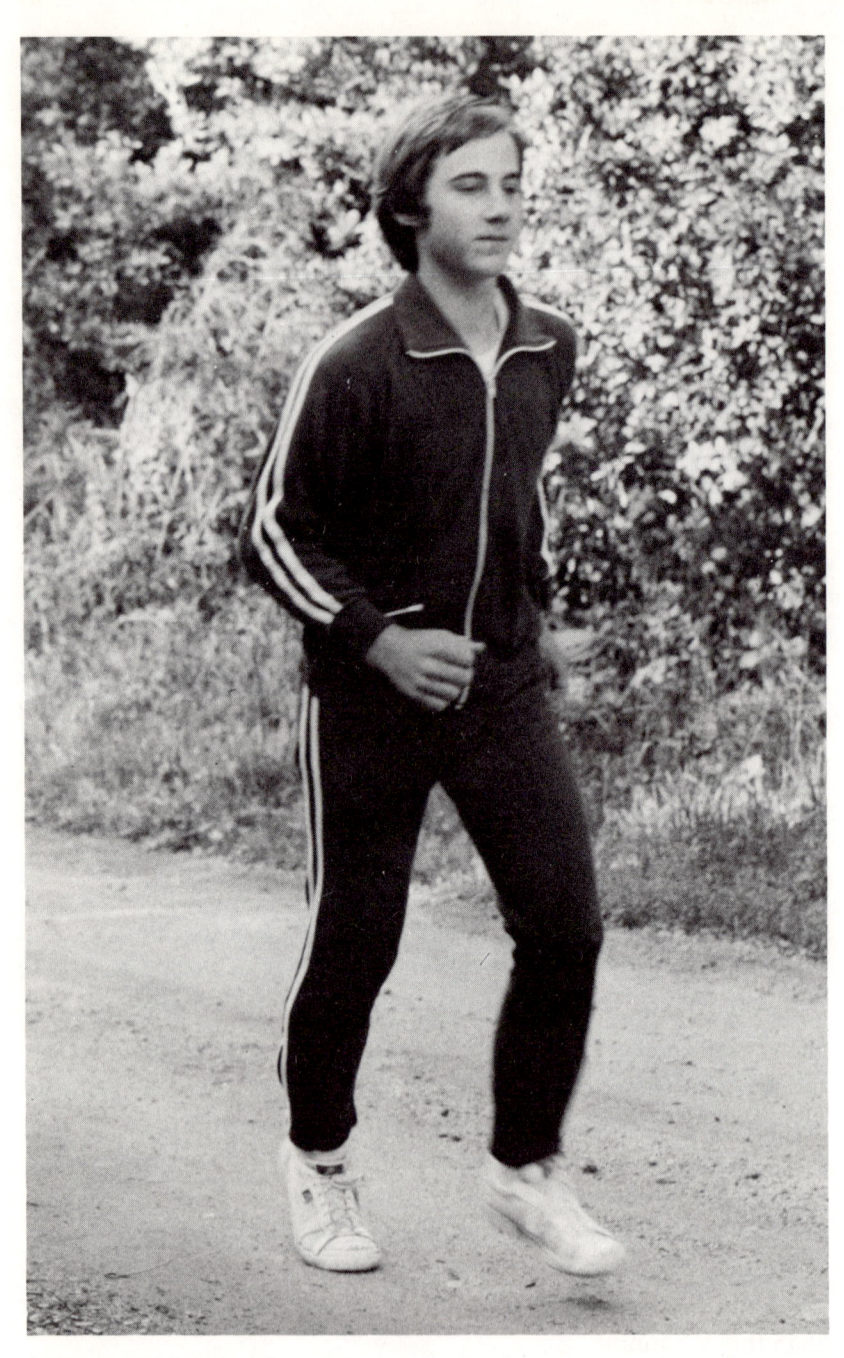

A country road is ideal for jogging, and just a few minutes a day will give you the aerobic training effect you need.

Dr. Cooper's point system, jogging a mile at a five-mile-an-hour clip is worth two points. At six miles an hour it is worth three points. Running the distance at seven-and-a-half miles an hour is worth four points. If you can run a six-and-a-half-minute mile, you can earn six points.

This is one reason why jogging and running have become so popular. You can earn all the aerobic points you need in just a few minutes. Many joggers and runners actually follow an every-other-day schedule, spending perhaps a half hour at heavy workouts Monday, Wednesday, and Friday, and doing just a few minutes of walking, stationary running, or rope skipping on the other days.

As you have undoubtedly seen, the jogger's garb follows no known dress code. You can wear whatever suits your taste and the weather. In summer, a T shirt and a pair of shorts will give both comfort and freedom. In winter, however, you will have to bundle up, but even in severe cold, you can stay relatively warm in long underwear, a sweat suit, gloves, and earmuffs or a cap that protects the ears.

Shoes for running and jogging must be selected with more attention than you give the rest of your outfit, particularly if you must run on hard surfaces. The jogger's most common complaint is sore feet. The most common cause is poor shoes with inadequate support and padding. Cheap canvas sneakers with thin soles are not adequate for hard surfaces. The extra money you spend for a pair of good jogging shoes with well-padded rubber or neolite soles will be money well spent.

Jogging and running styles vary a great deal, but there are a few things you should avoid. Don't look down at your feet. Hold your head up. At the same time don't lean back with a sway-back posture. Let your body lean forward at an angle that is natural for you. Your arms should swing freely. They control your pace. Force them to swing faster and you will run faster.

Legs should swing freely from the hips. With jogging, your knees will usually be slightly bent with ankles limber when your leading foot hits the ground. Runners often straighten the leg fully to extend their stride. Joggers, however, call this "overstriding."

Runners and joggers like to use foot-strike to describe styles.

Heel-to-toe foot-strike means that the heel of your leading foot hits the ground first. Then, as your body passes over the foot, it rocks forward so that the toe is the last point of contact.

The flat-footed strike lacks this rocking motion. You land with the entire foot and lift heel and toe at the same time. With the ball-of-the-foot strike, your heel does not touch the ground until your body is passing over the foot. Sprint runners usually stay up on the balls of their feet through the entire stride, but this is too tiring for distant running.

For those long distances, the heel-to-toe strike is probably better than the flat-footed strike, but you need not be too concerned about this at the beginning. Develop the style that comes naturally to you.

When you begin jogging or running, you may develop sore ankles. This is a fairly common complaint among beginners. Modify your program. Instead of jogging or running, take daily walks for a week or two. Then mix jogging with walking, and gradually ease back to a full session of jogging or running.

Shin splints or buck shins are another hazard, caused usually by hard surface or downhill running. This discomfort is due to a slight tear in the connective tissue along the front of the shin bone. It is not serious, but it can be very painful, forcing you to follow a modified program for several days. If you are prone to shin splints, you should at least give up running down hills. It's not very wise in any case. Give yourself a breather and walk until your route levels off again.

SWIMMING

If you have access to a pool, you can take up one of the best, perhaps the best, single fitness activities in the world. Swimming stretches and flexes all major muscle systems of the body, and it gives prompt returns in aerobic training effect.

The returns vary somewhat according to the stroke you use. Dr. Cooper found that the breaststroke requires the least oxygen consumption, seven millimeters per kilogram of body weight per minute. The backstroke is next with eight, followed closely by the overhand crawl, with nine. The butterfly takes the most oxygen, twelve millimeters per kilogram of body weight per minute.

His point ratings are based on the overhand crawl. They show that swimming this style for 200 yards in five minutes will earn one point. If you speed up, approaching a time of three minutes and twenty seconds, you will earn a point-and-a-half. Covering the distance in less than three minutes and twenty seconds will earn two-and-a-half points. When you can increase your distance to 600 yards and swim it in less than fifteen minutes, you will be earning five points. Doing this six times a week will give thirty points.

If you cannot achieve this pace, you can still earn your necessary points by extending your distance. For instance, covering 800 yards in less than twenty-six-and-a-half minutes will also earn five points.

CYCLING

In the past decade the bicycle has been rediscovered, and thousands of people, young and old, have taken to the sport. It is not only good recreation, but it is also a practical means of transportation. In addition, cycling leads to aerobic fitness.

Covering two miles in eight to twelve minutes is worth a point on Dr. Cooper's rating charts. Cut your time below eight minutes and you earn two points. Speed up to do two miles in less than six minutes, and it's worth three points.

When you can pedal four miles in less than twelve minutes—a twenty-mile-an-hour pace—you will earn six points. Do that five times a week, and you will be earning your thirty points.

Terrain and wind conditions must be considered in rating your effort, but normally, if you pick a loop route, these factors balance out.

Cycling on wet pavement is risky, and when ice or snow is on the streets, you should not go out at all. There are racks on the market that will convert your bike into an exercycle for indoor work. Of course, an exercycle itself will answer the same need, and most exercycles come with gauges and wheel loading devices that allow you to measure and control your effort.

SPORTS

Handball, squash, basketball, soccer, lacrosse, and hockey all have high aerobic ratings. Twenty minutes of continuous action at any of these sports is worth three points. Wrestling produces an even higher training effect. A tough, ten-minute match is worth four points.

Rowing also has a high yield. Eighteen minutes of two-oar rowing with a pace of twenty strokes a minute is worth four points.

Twenty minutes of evenly matched singles in tennis or badminton will give one-and-a-half points. Twenty minutes of fencing yields two points. Thirty minutes of snow skiing, water skiing, or football yields three points. Thirty minutes of ice skating, roller skating, or volleyball is worth two points.

Eighteen holes of golf is worth three points provided you do not use a motorized cart.

The big problem with sports is that you rarely maintain a continuous pace. Action slows down. There is dead time between plays. There are timeouts. In team sports, positions also make a big difference. A goalkeeper in soccer or hockey, for instance, will usually get more aerobic benefit from team practice sessions than he will in an actual game.

FURTHER READING

The aerobic phase of your program is so important that you will profit from more detailed knowledge on the training effect and how to achieve it. Dr. Cooper writes with great enthusiasm on his theories and his findings. Two of his books, *Aerobics* and *The New Aerobics,* both available in paperback from Bantam Books, give detailed charts with point ratings for all the exercises listed in this chapter. The charts are particularly helpful in planning a step-by-step program that will eventually lead to a thirty-point goal.

A different approach to the ratings of aerobic exercises is offered by Dr. Laurence E. Morehouse and Leonard Gross in *Total Fitness,* published by Pocket Books. Dr. Morehouse relates training effect with pulse rate, an approach that makes it possible to make your own evaluations of aerobic exercises.

Part Three *Supplementals*

8 *Stretch with Yoga*

There are so many different Yoga exercises that it is difficult to point to typical traits that distinguish them from other exercises. As a general rule, however, most Yoga positions involve a balance of dynamic forces, a give and take of muscles and joints.

Yoga rarely involves continuous motion. You take a specific position, hold it usually for ten to twenty slow counts and then release the position. By taking the same position just two or three times in one session, you will get full benefit from the exercise.

The benefits include both flexing and stretching, but generally the stretching is what you feel the most. The exercises in this chapter, which will introduce you to Yoga, were selected primarily for the strong stretching benefits they produce.

You should try all these exercises, but you will probably work just a few of them into your daily program. This does not mean that you should not change your pattern from day to day and week to week. This will give your workouts variety and give you added incentive. Yoga is not easy. Mastering an exercise brings a great sense of satisfaction and well-being.

If nothing else, this chapter should break down any prejudice you may have toward these ancient exercises. Unfortunately, too many Westerners tend to discount the wisdom of the East. They particularly suspect foreign philosophies and religions.

Don't get the idea that you have to change your religion to enjoy Yoga. You don't have to meditate or chant magic words. The exercises speak for themselves. They will do you a world of good, and it does not matter where in the world you come from.

Let's begin with the exercises designed to benefit what Yoga practitioners believe is the body's most important region.

THE BACK

We were all born with flexible spines, but few of us retain this flexibility. As we age, our backs stiffen. Yoga can reverse the stiffening process.

The Yoga Bend. Stand with your feet together and your legs straight. Bend forward from the waist as low as possible and clasp your hands behind your legs. Use your arms to pull your chest toward your thighs, your head toward your knees. Now slide your hands lower down. If you can get them below your calves, you will be off to a good start. Pull with your arms again and hold the position for a count of ten. Unless you are already very limber, you will bend your knees when you begin performing this exercise. Don't let a slight knee bend concern you. The main purpose here is to extend the spine. Later, you will be able to keep the knees straight and get the bonus benefit of a good stretch in the back of the legs.

Leg Pull. Sit with your legs stretched out and your feet together. Place your hands on your knees, let your body relax. Slowly lift your arms in a graceful arc. Stretch them high above your head and continue the motion until your body is leaning back several inches, enough to make your abdominal muscles flex. Now come forward slowly. Let your upper body relax so its own weight carries it forward. Now grip your calves with your hands and bend your elbows out to pull with your arms. This will bring your head close to your knees. Hold this position for a count of five. Then slide your hands toward your ankles and pull again. Hold this new position for another count of five. Then return to the starting position with your hands on your knees and repeat the exercise two more times. If you stick with this exercise daily for a few weeks, the restrictive tension will melt from your back almost magically. You

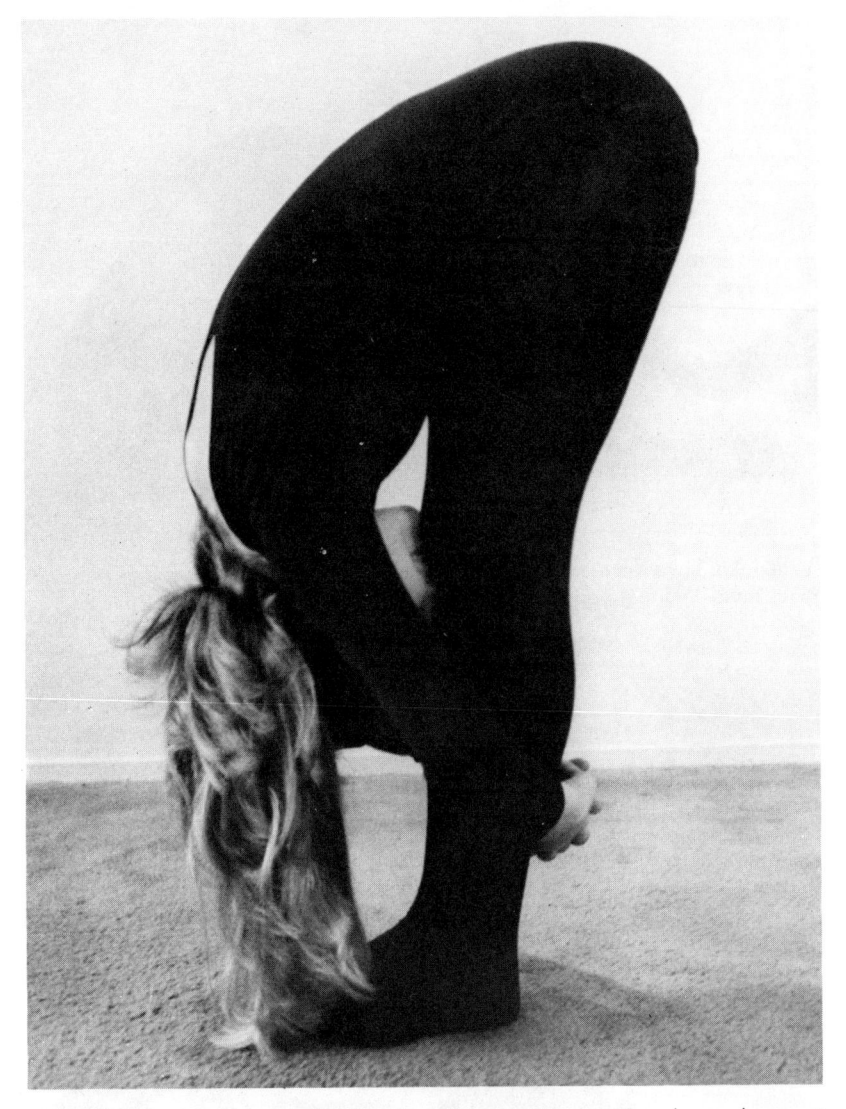

The Yoga bend is a wonderful stretcher. You may have to bend your knees at first, but with repeated, daily performance, your flexibility will increase quickly.

will be able to grip your ankles and rest your head on your knees. With continued work, you can achieve the advanced position—head resting on your knees and hands clasped below your feet.

The Bow. Like the cobra, described in Chapter 1, the bow develops reverse flexibility of the spine. This, however, is an ad-

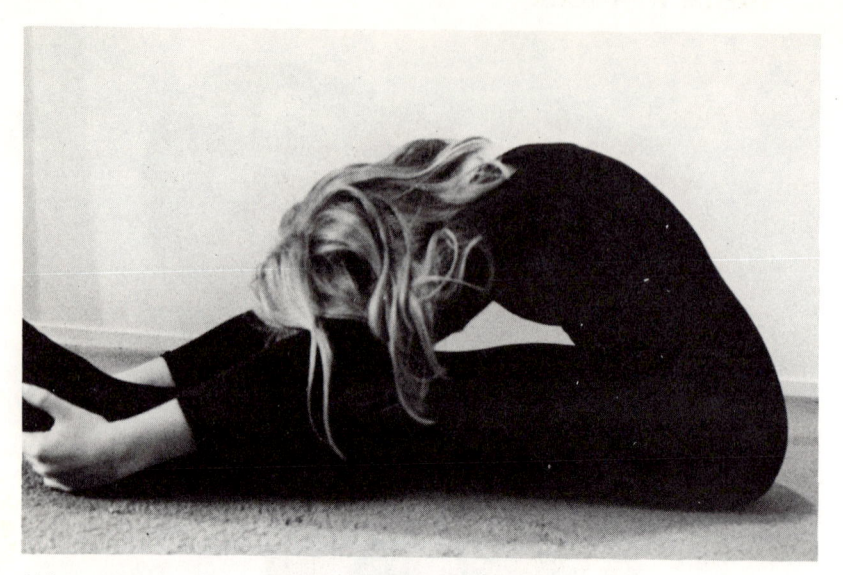

When you have developed good flexibility you can do advanced leg pulls with your hands holding your feet.

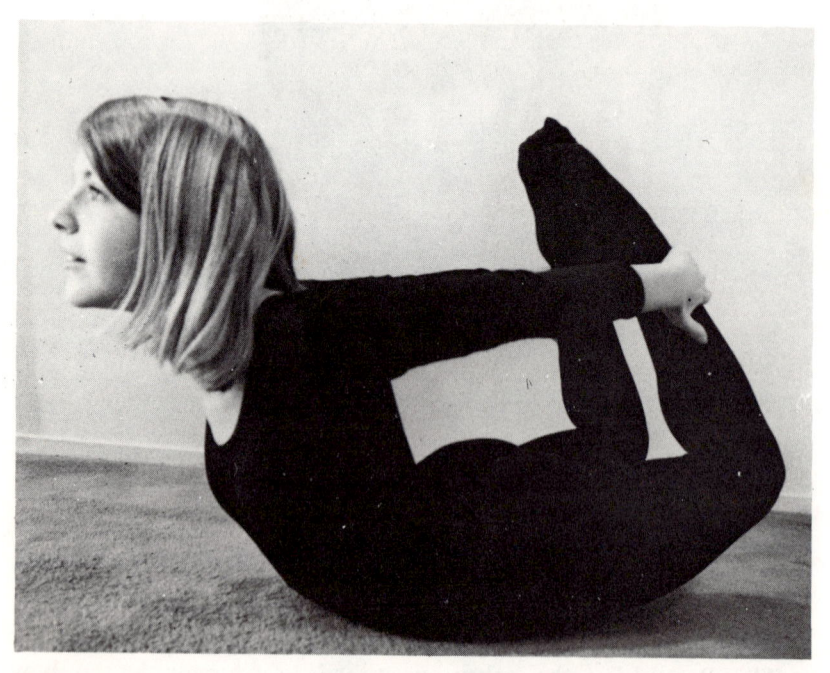

Powerful forces go to work in the bow. Develop reverse flexibility in the spine with the cobra before you advance to this exercise.

vance exercise with powerful force. Do not attempt it until after you have mastered the cobra. Lie on your stomach with your arms at your sides. Bend your knees, bringing your feet forward so that you can reach back and grip them firmly with your hands. Now pull with your arms so that you lift your upper trunk and your thighs from the floor. Bend your neck back toward your feet which should be well above your buttocks. If possible, hold the position for a count of ten. Do the bow twice each session. You must resist the tendency to hold your breath. There are special breathing exercises for advanced Yoga, but for these, stick to normal breathing.

The Twist. Just getting into position for the twist may be difficult at first, but once you master this exercise, you will be able to give the muscles in your lower back and your buttocks a good stretch. Begin in a sitting position with your legs outstretched. Bend your left leg and use your hands to tuck your left foot snug against your groin. Your left knee should be touching the floor. Now bend your right leg, bringing the knee up and swinging the foot out to place it on the floor just outside the left knee. You may have to prop your right hand behind you to keep from losing your balance during this maneuver. Next, grip your left knee with your left hand and place your right hand in the small of your back. Turn your upper trunk as far to the right as possible and hold the position for the count of ten. Face forward, rest a moment, and then repeat for another count of ten. Now, unwind and reverse your leg and arm positions for two more repetitions, twisting now to the left.

While all this may sound like the instructions for making a pretzel, the twist is well worth the effort.

The Plow. Lie on your back with your hands at your sides, palms down. Slowly raise your legs. Keep them straight together as you bring them up in a continuous arc. Soon after they pass the vertical position, lift your buttocks and lower back slowly from the floor. Continue moving your legs until your toes touch the floor above your head. Hold the position for the count of ten. Now move your legs slowly back to the vertical position. Bend your knees to a tuck, then straighten and lower them to the floor. Do the plow at least twice.

Move slowly, extending the vertibrae gradually from your lower

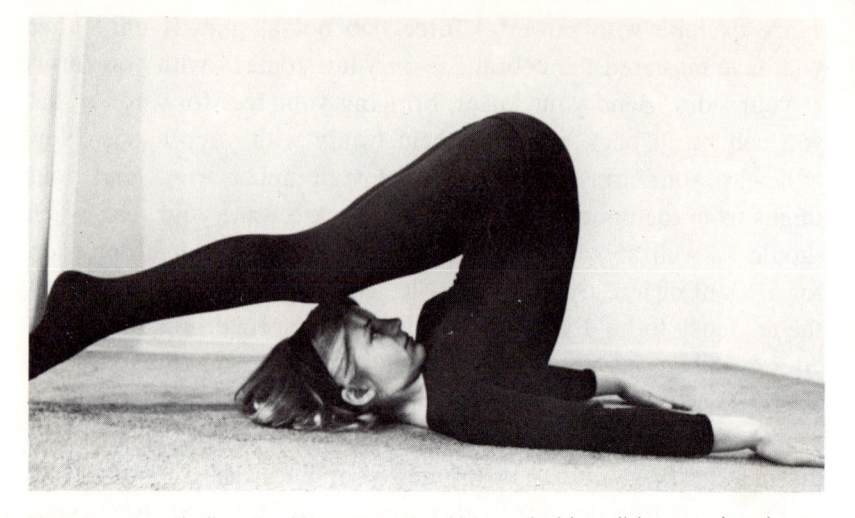

104   THE COMPLETE BEGINNER'S GUIDE TO PHYSICAL FITNESS

The plow is a challenging Yoga exercise. You probably will have to bend your knees at first, but when you gain flexibility, you will get tremendous satisfaction in performing the plow properly.

back to your shoulders. In the beginning, don't be concerned if you may have to bend your knees slightly before reaching the hold position.

LEGS

If you must spend much of your day sitting at a desk or bench, the following exercises will be particularly beneficial in working out the stiffness of leg muscle tension.

Alternate Leg Pulls. Sit on the floor with legs straight and feet together. Now bend your right leg, knee out and close to the floor. Bring your right heel up against the inside of your left thigh. Now reach up with hands extended. Lean backward a few inches before coming forward to clasp your hands around your left ankle. Now, with elbows out, gently pull your trunk forward as far as possible. Let your neck go limp. Hold the position for a count of twenty. Release your hold and straighten up. Repeat and then do the exercise twice again with leg position reversed.

Alternate leg pulls stretch muscles of the buttocks and upper thighs. After two or three weeks of leg pulls, you may be ready for

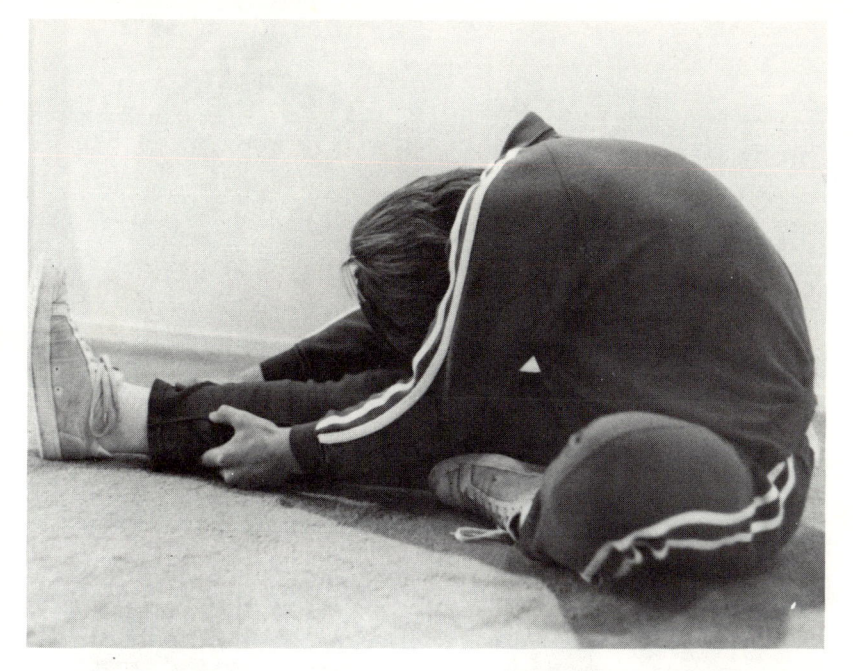

Alternate leg pulls should be held for a count of ten and repeated again at least once. Pull your body forward by cocking your elbows out.

advanced leg pulls. Here you clasp the foot instead of the ankle, and if possible rest your head on the knee of the extended leg.

The Bridge. Another real stretch for the back of the legs can be achieved with this exercise which begins on all fours. Knees should be together and hands about shoulder-width apart. Now straighten your legs, lifting your weight to your feet and hands. Arch your body as high as possible, but let your head hang low on a limp neck. Hold this position for a count of ten. Then inch your feet forward toward your head. Go as far as possible without bending your knees or lifting your hands. If possible, keep your heels on the floor. Hold this position for another count of ten.

Toe Twist. This exercise will strengthen your feet and ankles and improve balance. Stand with arms extended, palms down and thumbs touching. Keep your eyes on the backs of your hands. Now lift up on your toes and slowly turn your arms to the left, turning your trunk to follow until it is at a right angle with your feet. Hold

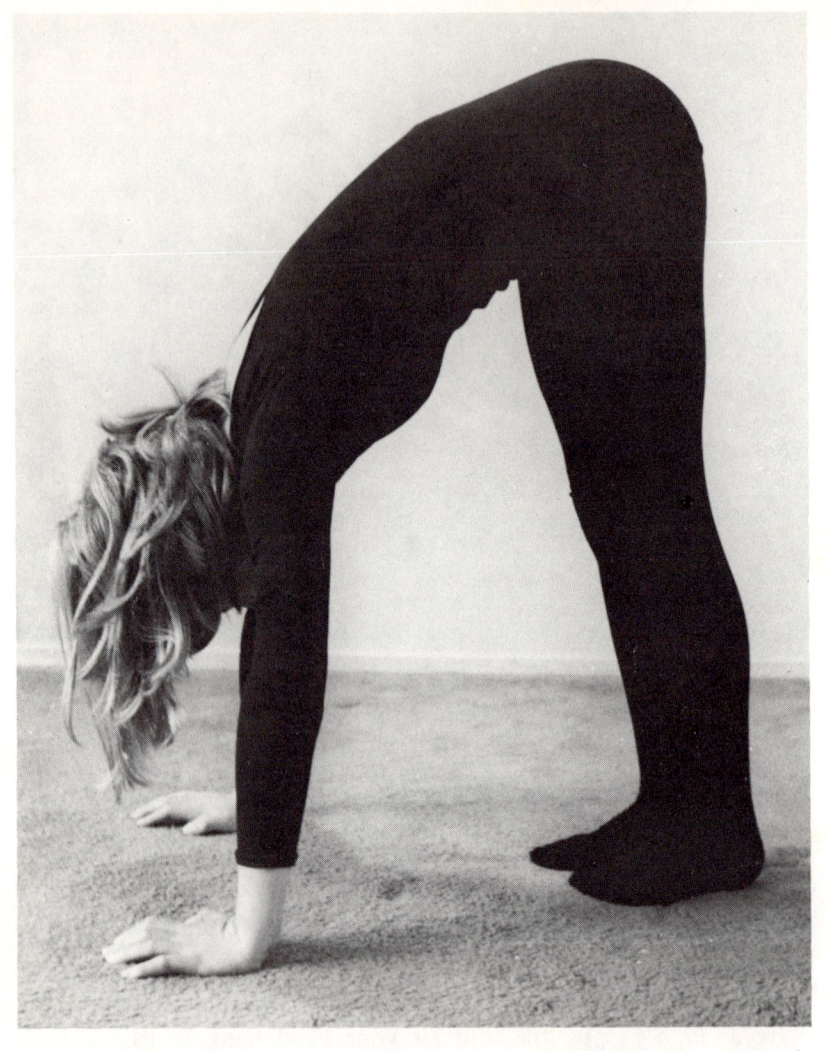

The bridge will give the muscles along the back of your legs a real stretch, particularly if you can keep your heels on the floor.

for a count of five. Then return slowly to the starting position. Now repeat, turning this time to the right. Perform this at least twice to each side. When you can do this smoothly with no jerky motions or shifting of feet, you have developed good body balance.

Thigh Stretch. This is a simple but effective exercise that limbers the knees and loosens thigh muscles. Sit on the floor with knees bent and open. Clasp your hands on your feet and draw them as

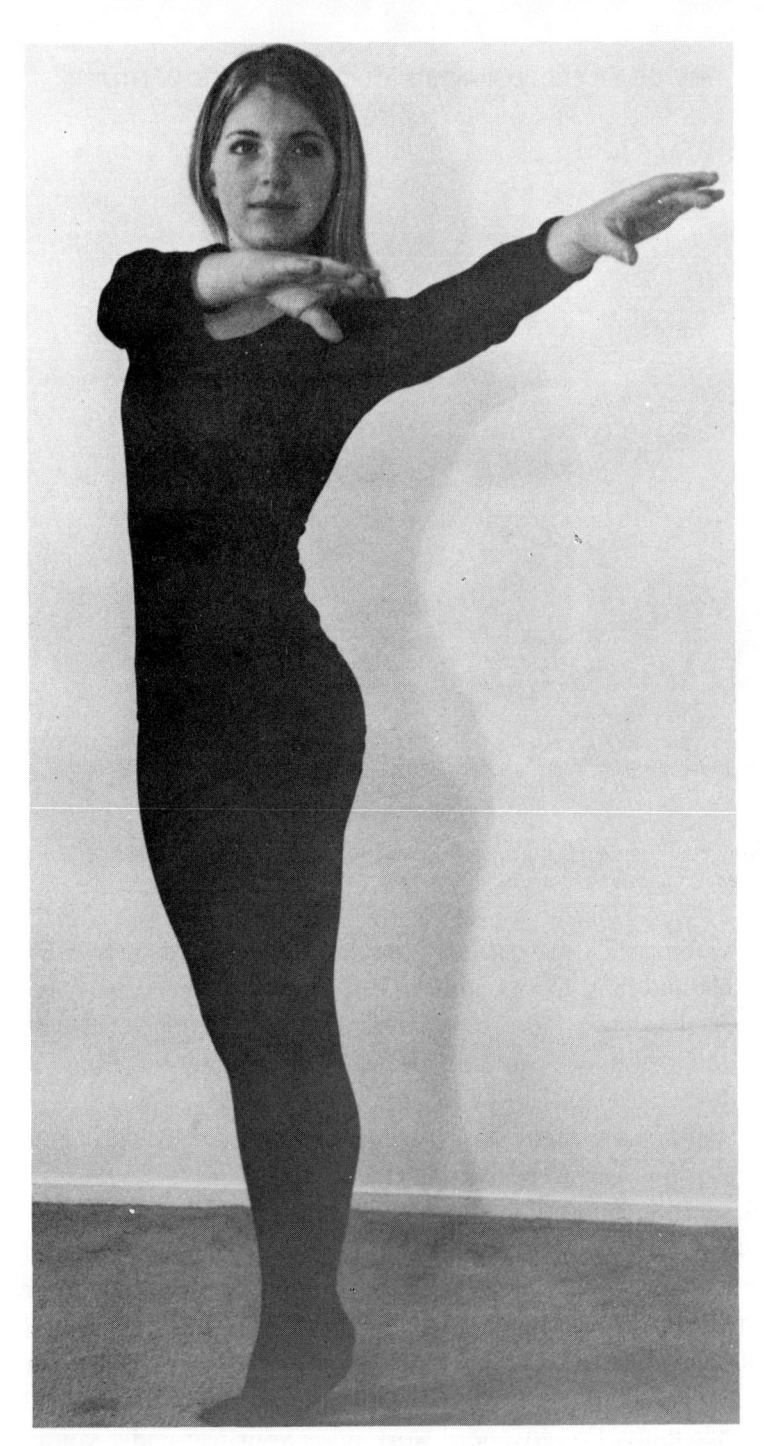

Yoga toe twist.

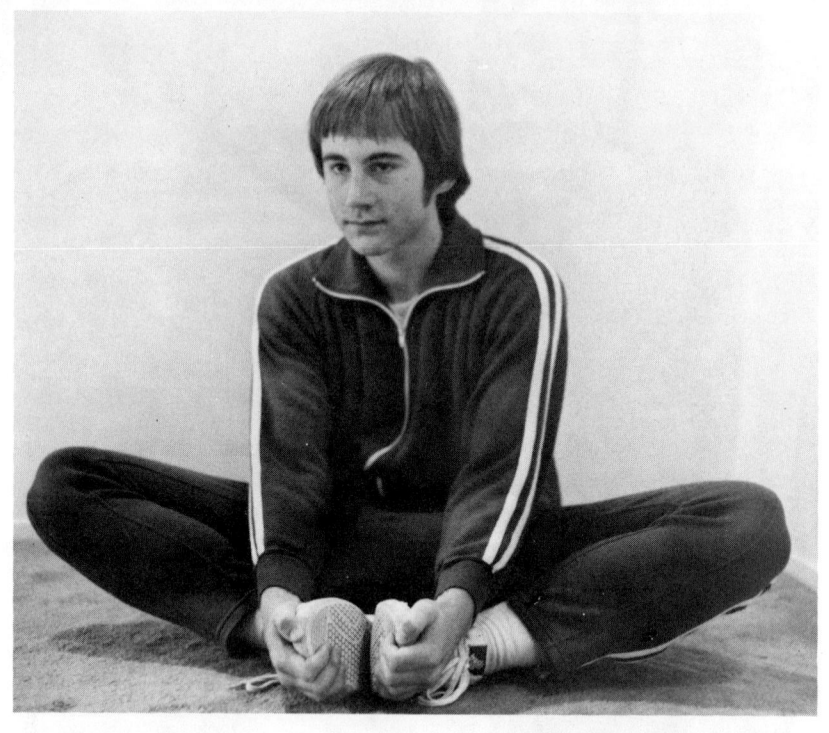

The thigh stretch is simple but effective. When you are limber, your knees will rest on the floor during your hold position.

close to your crotch as possible. Now let your knees drop as wide as possible and hold for a count of ten. Relax and then repeat the exercise at least two more times. Eventually, you will be able to achieve the advanced position with the knees actually touching the floor.

Back Bend. Like many Yoga exercises, this benefits the whole body, but it has special benefits for the feet and toes. Sit with your buttocks resting on your heels, toes together, pointing backward. Place your hands behind you so that you must lean backward at least thirty degrees. Lower your head and arch your back. Hold for a count of ten. Now slowly slide your hands back farther behind you and lean back as far as possible. Hold this position for another count of ten. Return to the starting position, rest a moment, and repeat once more. For advanced work place your feet under you in a vertical position so that your weight is on your toes and the balls of your feet.

STRETCH WITH YOGA

The Lotus. This is the position that most people think of on the first mention of Yoga. It limbers the knees, ankles, and feet as well as the thighs and buttocks.

Start with the half lotus. Place the left heel as close to the body as possible with the sole against the inside of the right thigh. Now bring the right foot up and place it on top of the left thigh close to the groin. Hold this for a full minute if possible. Then reverse the position of the legs and hold again.

For the full lotus, which you will be able to perform when your legs loosen up, the left foot is placed high on the right thigh and the right foot high on the left thigh. Both knees should touch the floor. Traditionally, the hands should rest on the knees with the thumb and forefinger touching. Eyelids should be lowered but not closed. The position does indeed encourage meditation.

Reverse the position of your legs, and practice the lotus until you can hold it at least a minute with no discomfort.

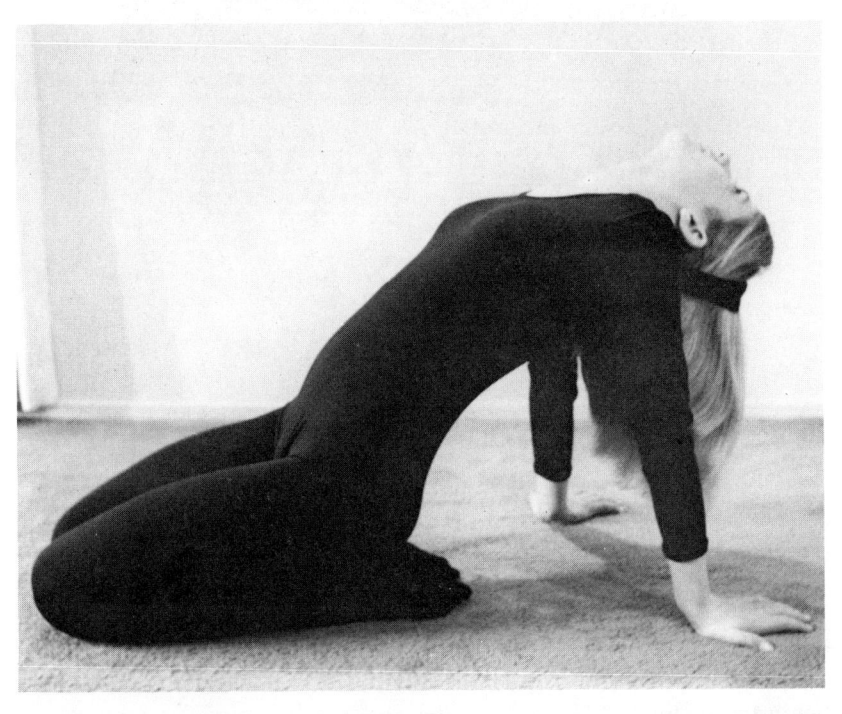

The back bend stretches many muscles, but your feet and ankles will receive the greatest benefit.

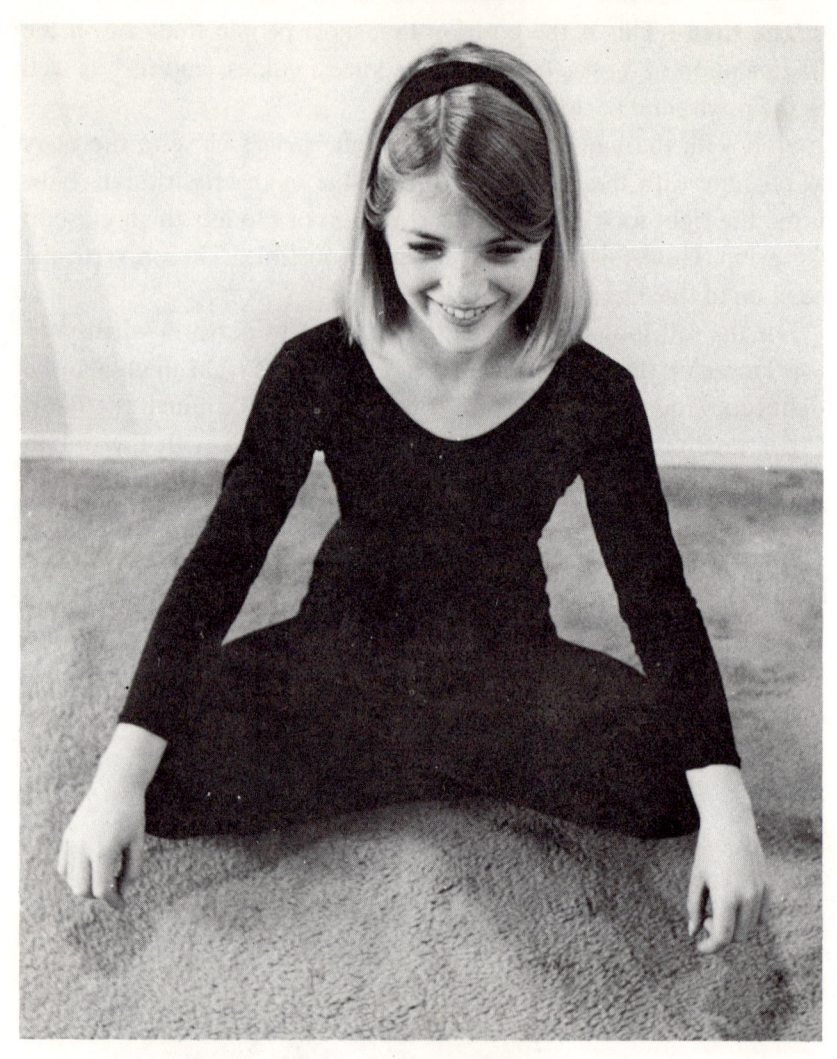

If you have trouble with the lotus position, start with the half lotus. Eventually, you should be able to hold the full lotus without discomfort for at least a minute.

NECK AND SHOULDERS

Shoulder Raise. This is particularly helpful for people who spend long hours at a desk. It takes the fatigue out of the upper back and shoulders. Sit in a lotus or half lotus position and clasp your hands behind your back. Very slowly straighten your arms and raise them behind you as high as possible. Hold the position for the count of five. Then lower the hands slowly. Repeat at least five times.

Neck Twist. You can do this when sitting at a table or desk or when lying on your stomach. It will loosen up a stiff neck and take away many of the general body tensions resulting from tension around the complex nerve network of the neck. Rest the elbows on the floor or desk and cover your ears with your palms. Your forearms should be almost parallel. Bend your neck forward and clasp your hands behind your head. Pull down until your chin rests on your chest. Hold for a count of ten.

Next, without moving your arms, lift your head and turn it to the left so that your chin is cupped in the palm of the left hand. Place your right hand on the back of your head, using it to turn the head as far to the left as possible. Hold for a count of ten. Then repeat, with the head turned right and the hand positions reversed. Hold again for a count of ten.

GRACE AND BALANCE

Because you do most Yoga exercises slowly, they lead naturally to grace and balance. A few exercises put special stress on these qualities, qualities that go hand in hand with good posture, body awareness, and general well-being.

Side Bends. Sitting in a lotus or half lotus position, clasp your hands behind your head. Keeping both knees on the floor, bend as far to the left as possible and hold the position for a count of five. When you are limber, you will be able to touch your elbow to the floor. Straighten up slowly. Now bend your body to the left and touch your right elbow to your left thigh. Again, hold for a count of five before coming up slowly. Repeat both movements in the other direction.

In addition to balance, these bends help tone the muscles of the waist and abdomen. They are best done in full lotus position.

Head Stands. Few people are able to stand on their heads with their first attempt. In Yoga you can start with a modified head stand. Begin on all fours. Lower your head to the floor and clasp your hands behind your head. Your elbows should be out with your forearms braced on the floor. Now straighten your legs and come up on your toes. Work your feet as close as possible toward your head and hold the position for a count of ten. Come out of the position slowly. Move your feet back, drop to your knees and then lift your head. You should be able to hold the modified head stand for at least a minute and work up to three minutes. It is good for circulation and has been known to cure some tension headaches.

The full head stand begins in the same way as the modified head stand. Make sure that your head and forearms make a firm base. From the tiptoe position, swing your body forward and at the same time bend and lift your legs. It is important to bend the knees to lower your center of gravity. Straighten your legs slowly only after you are certain of your balance. Hold the position for at least thirty seconds. Eventually, you will be able to hold a head stand for three minutes or more.

Come out of the position slowly, bringing the knees down toward your chest, and then lowering your toes to the floor. If balance is a problem, begin doing head stands against a wall.

Leg and Arm Raise. In a standing position, begin by raising your right arm while you slowly raise your left leg behind you. Bend the leg so that you can clasp your foot in your left hand. Now, with your right arm straight up and your left foot as high as possible, bend your neck back lifting your chin high. Hold this position for the count of five. Come out of it slowly and then repeat in the reversed position.

The spine and thighs get a good workout in this balancing exercise.

Shoulder Stand. This starts like the plow, but instead of swinging the legs all the way over to touch your toes to the ground, lift them to a vertical position. Lift your hands to the small of your back and brace your elbows on the floor so you can lift your hips in line with your legs. If possible, hold legs and hips vertically for three minutes. To come out of the position, bend the knees slightly and let the legs come down over the head as you put your arms flat at your sides. Gradually flatten your hips to the floor before you lower your legs.

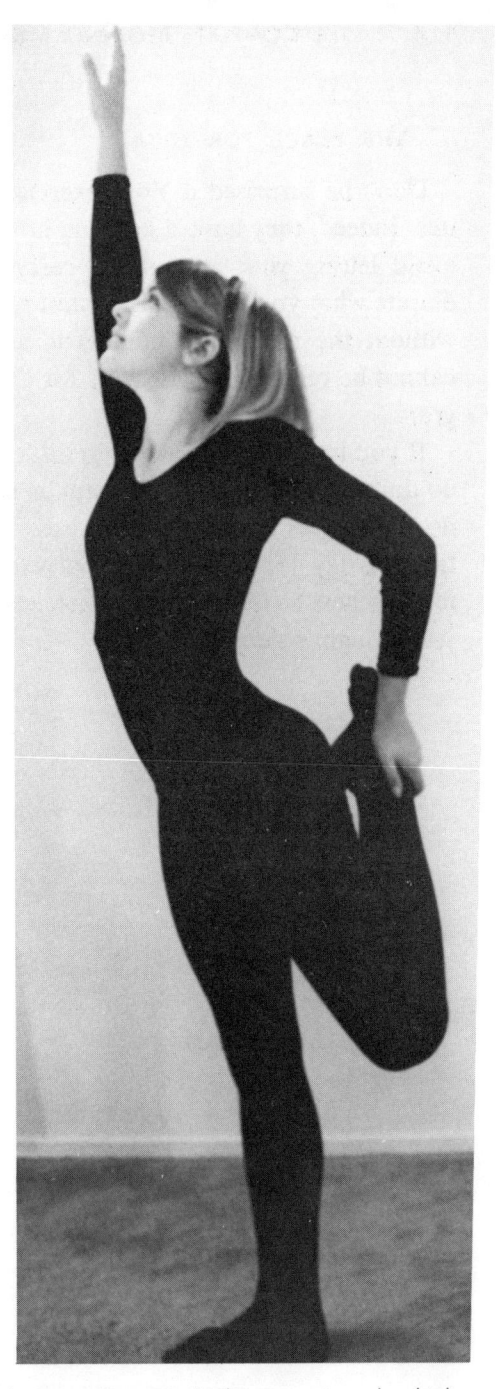

The leg and arm raise promotes balance and grace. At the same time, the thigh muscles get a good stretch.

THE PLACE FOR YOGA

Don't be surprised if Yoga exercises become your all-time favorites. Indeed, they have a growing host of enthusiastic followers, but avoid letting your enthusiasm carry you away completely. Yoga, despite what you may hear, cannot replace an aerobic exercise, and without the motion of miometric and pliometric exercises, Yoga cannot be relied on exclusively for the warm-up phase of your program.

If you find that there are several Yoga exercises that you want to do daily, use one or two of them as substitutes for pliometrics, but do the rest as additional exercises. You might set aside a special time of day for these additional exercises. You may discover, as many others have, that Yoga exercises just before bedtime lead to a restful night's sleep.

9 Isometrics

These exercises became very popular in the early 1950s, soon after German research on them was translated into English. German scientists claimed that isometrics—flexing without motion—could increase muscle size and strength by as much as 5 per cent a week.

That claim touched off an isometric craze, but subsequent research has modified the original claims substantially. Today, isometrics are the subject of much criticism and debate.

Dr. Cooper believes the static flexing of isometrics makes no significant increase in the muscles' demand for oxygen. He dismisses isometrics as a good way to develop muscles for performing isometrics and little else.

The exercises, however, do have real value in physical therapy, particularly when patients are immobilized by casts. Muscle tissue in such cases can be maintained by static flexing. Astronauts have used isometrics when other exercises in a weightless environment were impossible.

Many athletes use isometrics to build up certain sets of muscles even though the value of isometrics for sports conditioning is highly debatable. Several football teams have recently discarded isometric training programs when they were followed by an increase in injuries, particularly knee injuries.

Despite all the controversy, there is no doubt that isometrics do increase muscle size and probably contribute to increased strength. They have a place in your fitness program if you are anxious to gain weight in a hurry and want to be sure that you add muscle tissue and not fat tissue. But they should be done with moderation and should always be used as a supplement to pliometrics, miometrics, and aerobic workouts.

Performed properly, the flex in isometrics should be built up gradually and maximum flex should usually be held just briefly. The general rule is four seconds for build-up and six seconds for hold.

Since they are so brief, you can perform most of these exercises just about any time and any place. And you need no special equipment.

THE ABDOMEN

Lean-aways. Sit on the floor with knees bent and feet braced under a heavy piece of furniture. Lean back so that your head is just a few inches off the floor. Hold this position as long as possible. Rest and repeat once again. It is easiest to do this with your hands on your stomach. You can feel those muscles tighten. To make it tougher, clasp your hands behind your head.

This is the one exercise in this group that will produce benefit from an extended flex. For this reason some claim it is not truly an isometric exercise. There is no doubt, however, of its benefit in building the abdominals.

Pull-ins. Suck in your stomach as far as possible and hold for six seconds. It's as simple as that. You can do this any time, when you're walking, waiting for a bus, sitting at a desk, taking a shower. You can perform pull-ins in various positions. You can stand with your hands in the small of your back and pull in as if you wanted to touch your hands with the wall of your stomach. You can bend over with your hands placed just above your knees and pull in your stomach as you push down with your hands. Or you can sit in a chair, pulling on the sides of the chair seat with your hands as you pull in your stomach.

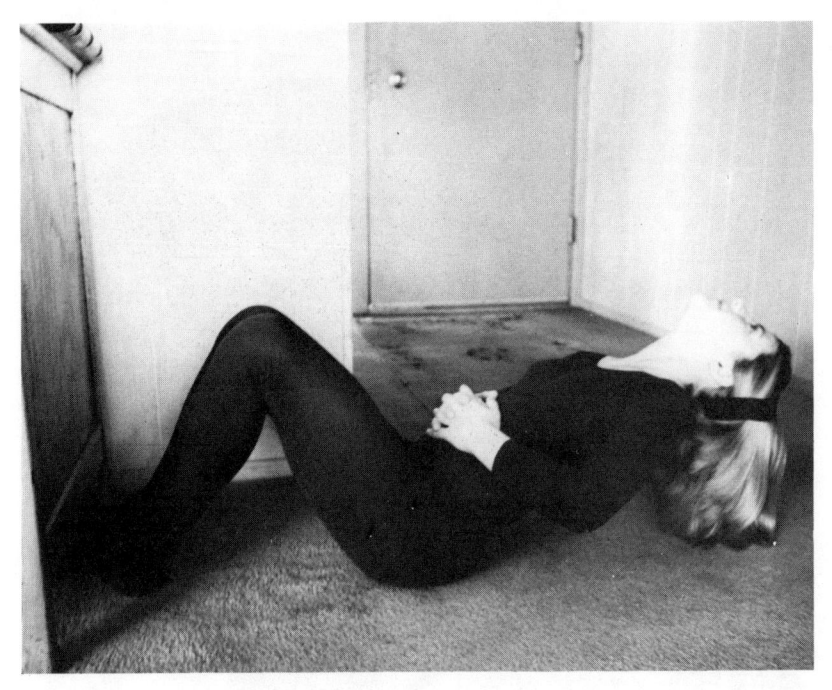

Lean-aways harden the abdominal muscles. In this position, you can feel the flex. For advanced work, however, you may want to hold your hands behind your neck.

Pull-ins, in fact, can be done while you perform many of the exercises described in earlier chapters.

LEGS AND HIPS

Tight Seat. Flex the buttock muscles. You can do this in any position, sitting, standing, even while walking. An old punishment in the French Army called for offenders to march around the parade ground holding a coin in the cleft of their flexed buttocks. Don't you try this prolonged penny pinching. Just flex and hold for six seconds and then repeat once.

When walking, try a pull-in at the same time you flex your buttocks. This promotes good posture.

Knee Pushes. There are various ways to try straightening your knees against resistance. The simplest is to do a bend-over with

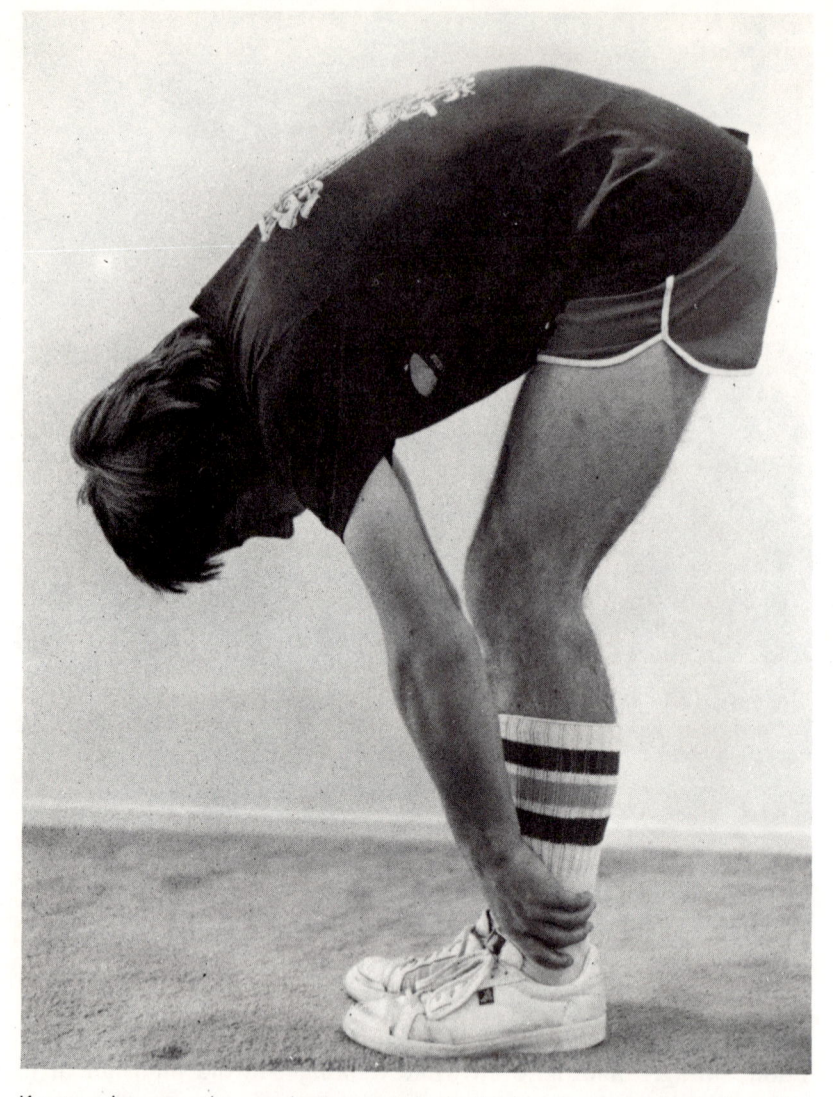

Knee pushes give the muscles up and down the legs a strong, static flex. You can get similar benefit working inside an open doorway, leaning against one jamb while pressing a foot against the other.

knees slightly bent. Grip your ankles firmly with your hands and then flex to straighten your knees.

This is so close to the Yoga bend described in the last chapter that you can shift from Yoga to isometrics with just a slight change of hand position.

ISOMETRICS

In an open doorway, you can do knee pushes by bracing your back against one jamb and putting a foot against the other, about level with your stomach. Push and hold for six seconds. Then repeat with the other leg.

Knee Presses. Sit in a chair with your knees about shoulder-width apart. Cup your left hand against the inside of your right

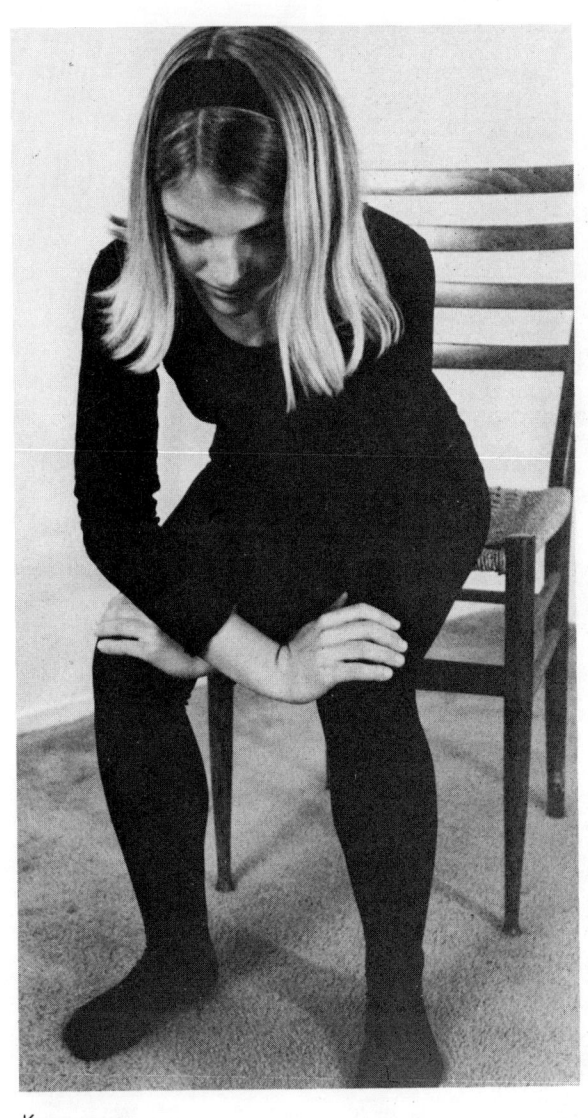

Knee press.

knee and your right hand against the inside of your left knee. Now try to press your knees together against the resistance of your hands.

Next, slide your hands over so they cup the outside of your knees. Try to force your knees apart against the pull of your hands.

Foot Presses. Sit forward on a chair so that your legs are straight

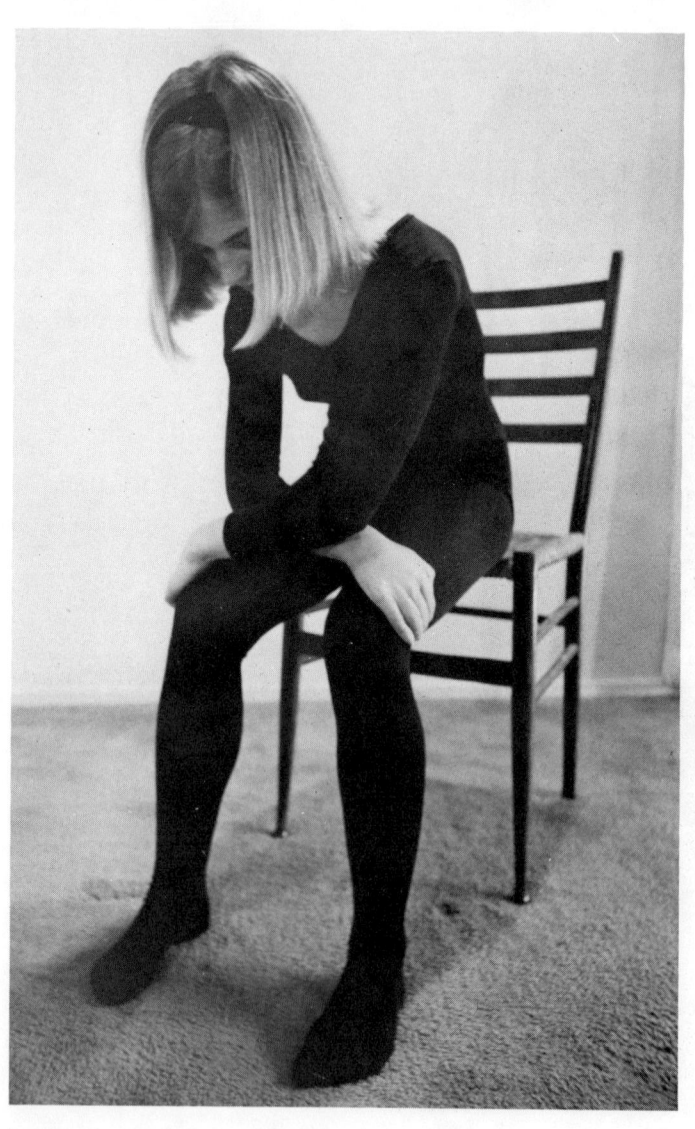

Reverse knee press.

ISOMETRICS

and your feet are on the floor about two feet apart. Flex your legs as if you were trying to squeeze a solid object between your feet. If you can't do this without bringing your feet together, put something, such as a stout wastebasket or a bucket, between your feet for this exercise.

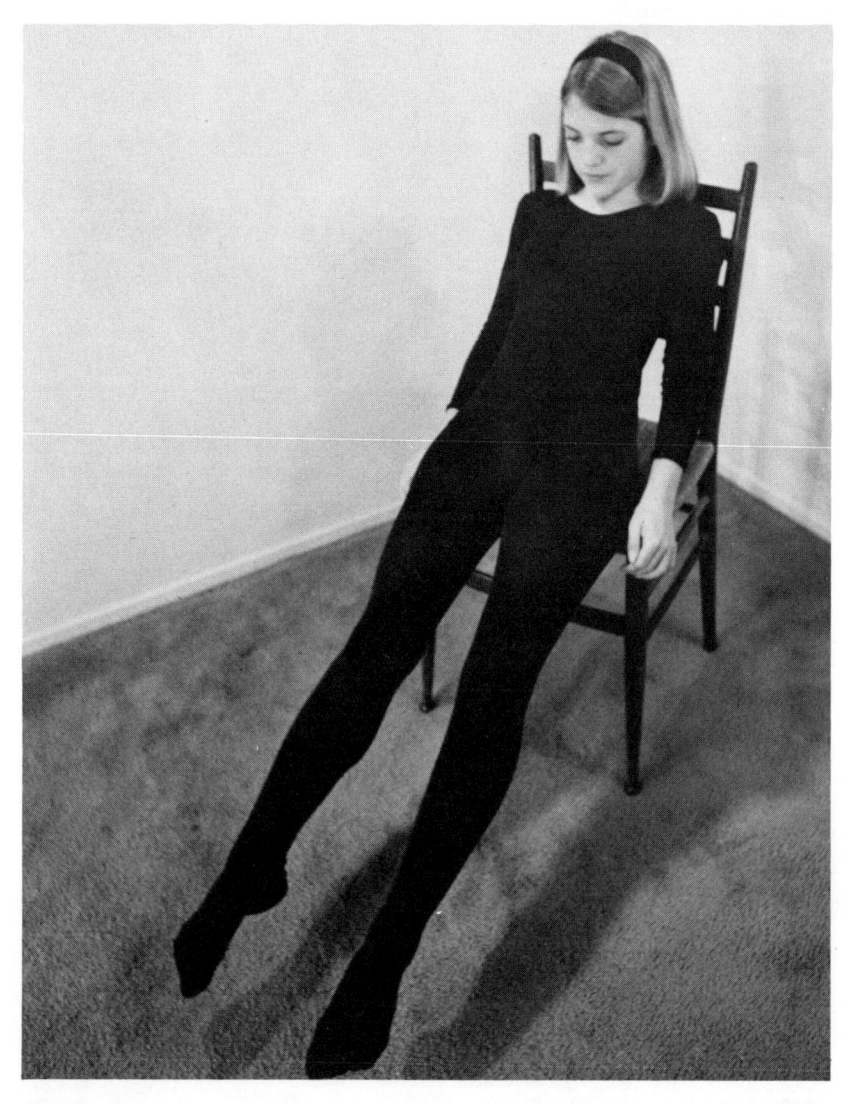

Foot press.

ARMS AND CHEST

Hand Lifts. Place one palm on top of the other at about waist level. Try to lift the lower hand as you press down with the upper hand. Switch hand positions and repeat. When sitting at a desk or heavy table, place your hands palm up beneath the desk or table top and try to lift.

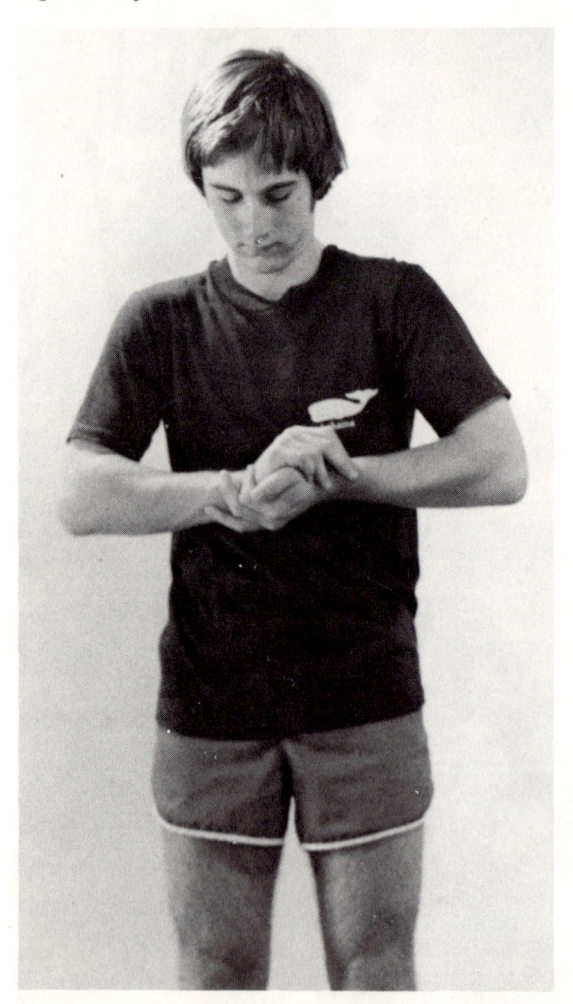

Hand lifts can be done at any level from waist to chest high. You can get the same benefit from placing the hands beneath a desk or other heavy piece of furniture and flexing to lift.

ISOMETRICS

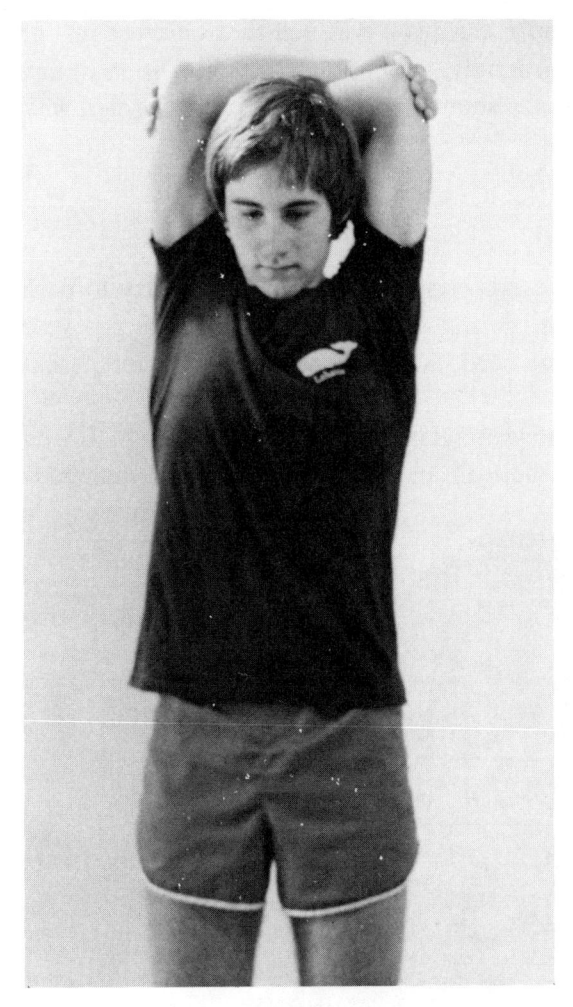

One form of arm pull calls for overlapping the forearms over the head and flexing to pull the arms apart.

Arm Pulls. Join your arms above your head so that your hands are cupped over your elbows. Try to pull your arms apart. Now hook your fingers together above your head and try to pull your hands apart. Next hold your clasped hands before you at chest level and pull. Now try it at waist level.

Arm Pushes. Overlap your hands so that one palm presses against the other. Flex to put full pressure on your palms. Do this with the hands at chest level and then at waist level. As you change level with arm pulls and presses you will find that different sets of muscles are affected. Generally, the chest muscles get the most flex with hands low, while the shoulder muscles get the most flex with hands high.

NECK AND BACK

Head Presses. With hands clasped on your forehead, try to push against their resistance, flexing the neck forward. Now put your hands at the back of the head, and push by flexing the neck backward.

You can do head presses against a wall or door jamb. If you stand a few feet from the wall and lean against it with your body

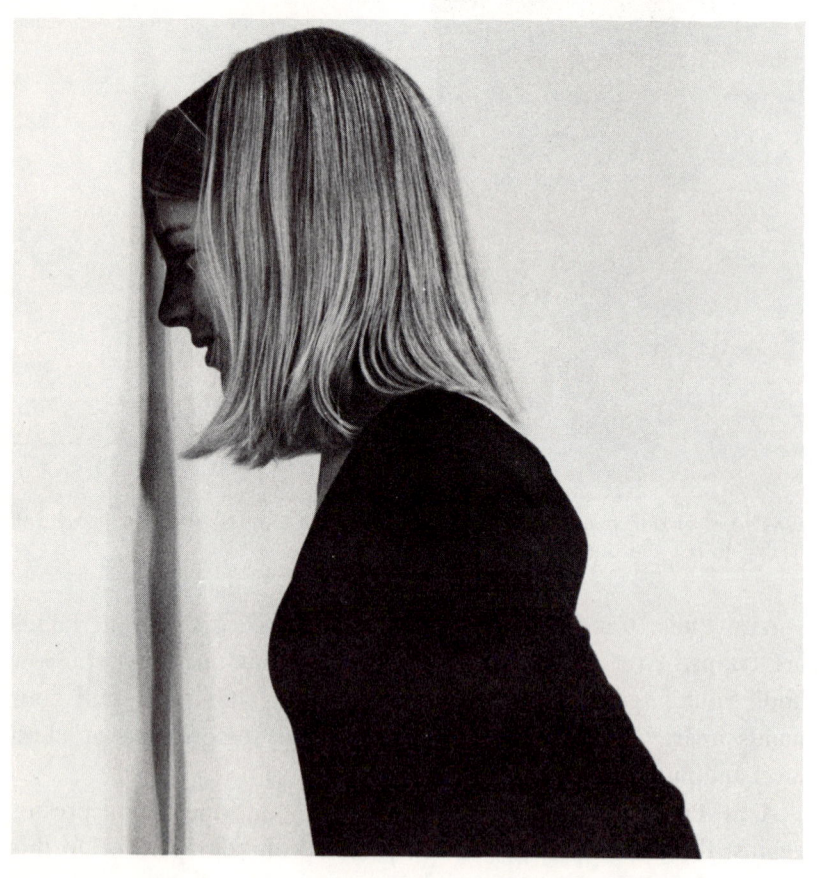

Head press against a wall.

ISOMETRICS 125

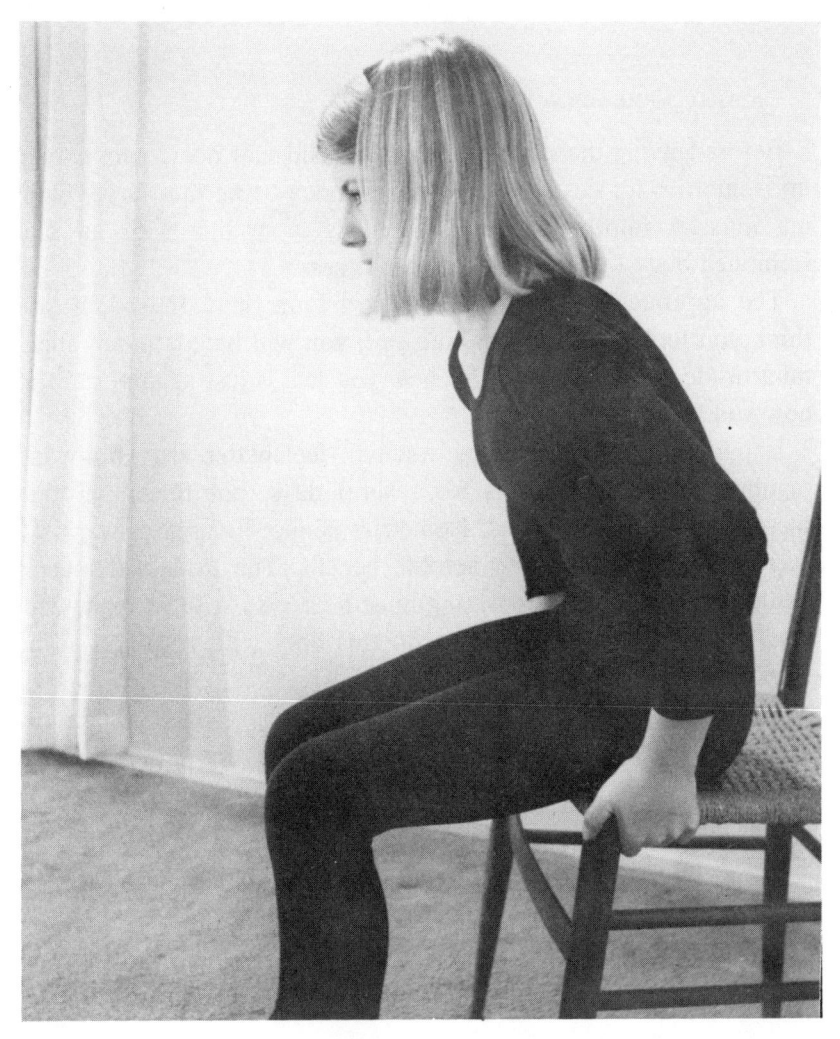

Sitting lifts with elbows cocked out and back bent will give the back and shoulder muscles a strong, static flex.

stiff, you will have good resistance for this flex. You can use your hands to cushion your forehead and the back of your head.

Sitting Lifts. Sit on the floor, hugging your knees tightly to your chest and try to straighten your spine. Sit in a chair and grip the sides of the seat with your elbows cocked so that your back is bent forward. Try to straighten your back without straightening your arms.

ABOUT APPEARANCE

Before leaving the subject, it must be said that many people take up isometrics for cosmetic reasons, the idea being that large, bulging muscles improve their looks. This is in line with an old-fashioned body-building approach to fitness.

The approach will be with us for a long time. Indeed, if you think you look good in a bathing suit, you will have a happy mental attitude about yourself. But how you feel is just as important as how you look.

Experiences differ. Perhaps you will feel better after following regular isometric workouts for several days, but remember that there is no motion involved. Isometrics cannot be used as warm-up exercises. And there is no aerobic benefit. The expanded muscle tissue you add with static flexing must be served with an expanded, healthy blood stream. You can do this only with regular aerobic workouts.

Some who have taken up isometrics have complained after a few weeks of sore muscles, even muscle spasms. If this should happen to you, cut the exercises from your program completely. Your particular muscle system is simply not designed for static flexing.

10 *Weights*

If you want to work with weights, you must be sure to recognize the difference between weight lifting and weight training.

Weight lifting is a competitive sport where the participants—grouped by body-weight classes—try to lift as much as they can. You should not take up weight lifting without expert supervision. This cannot be overemphasized. There have been far too many tragic injuries with weights, particularly among young people.

Competing or simply trying to show off with weights can lead to broken bones, torn ligaments or tendons, and ripped cartilage. These can be crippling injuries.

Weight training is conditioning with weights. There is no competition involved. In fact, with weight training the number of times you can repeat an exercise is a far more important measure of progress than the amount of weight you can lift. Weight training is a legitimate supplement to physical fitness. Coaches use it to prepare players for team sports, particularly hockey, baseball, and football. And a weight-training program is excellent for people who want to gain weight.

This is not to say that you must avoid weight lifting as a competitive sport. Youngsters, both boys and girls, can and do take it up, but they do it under the close supervision of a qualified instructor.

Even the most avid boosters of the sport warn against unsupervised weight lifting for anyone under sixteen years of age.

No matter what your goal, you should begin with weight training. The introductory exercises described below are for dumbbells of two to five pounds and barbells of ten pounds. Again, the number of repetitions you begin with should be a matter of personal judgment. But, as with any other exercise, you should try to increase your limits.

BARBELL EXERCISES

Snatch. Stand behind the barbell with feet about a foot apart. Keeping your back straight, bend your knees in a crouch as if you were sitting in a chair. Grip the bar with knuckles forward and hands about shoulder-width apart. Now straighten the legs forcefully to start the lift. Keep the bar close to you as you lift it all the way to the overhead position. Cock your wrists back when your arms are fully extended to give the bar firm support. Now lower the bar gradually, first to the chest with elbows bent. Then to the thighs with arms straight. And finally to the floor with knees bent in the same sitting posture you took at the start of the lift.

This is a good warm-up exercise for weight training. The impetus for the lift comes from the legs. Straighten them as if you were forcing your feet through the floor. This will start the bar up briskly so that your arms can complete the lift with little strain.

Two-hand Curl. Stand with your feet about shoulder-width apart and the bar held at thigh level with knuckles toward you. Keeping elbows tucked close to your body, lift the bar to your chest. This should be done with a slow movement of the forearms alone. Don't swing the bar up or let your body sway. The biceps will do most of the work both in raising the bar and in lowering it again slowly to your thighs.

Clean and Press. Stand behind the bar as you did for the snatch. Grip it with knuckles forward. Lift the bar to your shoulders, again letting your legs do most of the work. At the peak of your lift, your wrist should be cocked back so that your forearms come beneath the bar. The bar should rest lightly against the chest. This is the clean.

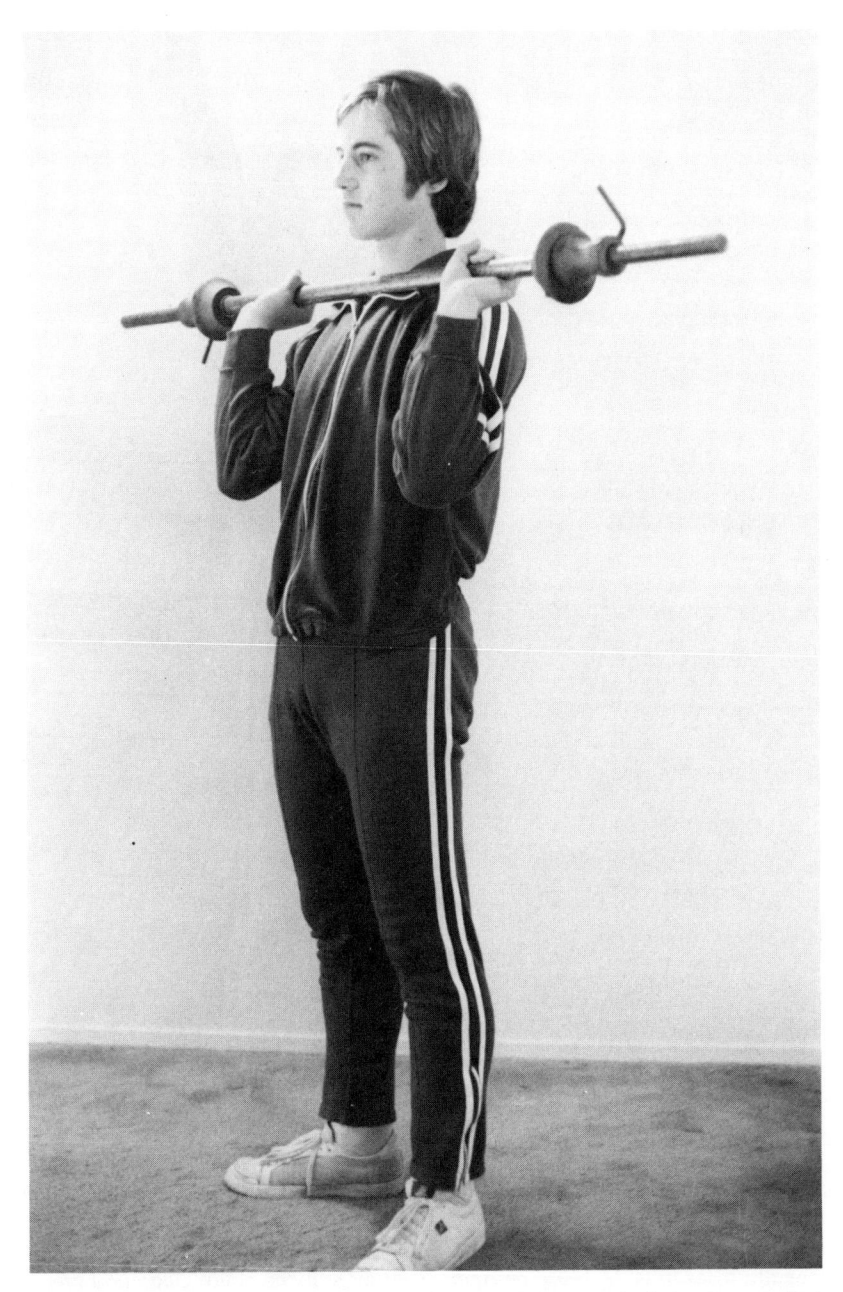

In the clean position, the bar should be at chest level with the wrists cocked to bring the forearms under the weight.

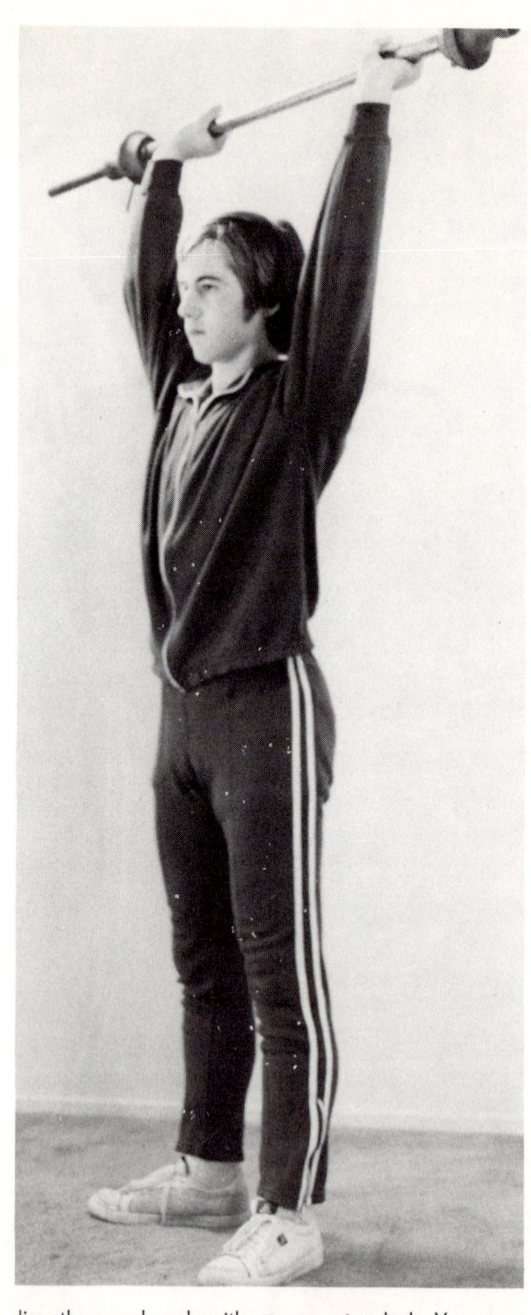

The press brings the bar directly overhead with arms extended. You can repeat presses from the clean position, or go through the entire clean and press for your repetitions.

WEIGHTS

Now you are ready to start the press. Lift the bar with smooth motion above the head. Pause for a moment with arms fully extended. Now lower the bar to the clean position. You can repeat presses from the clean position, or you can repeat the full clean and press. If you have difficulty cocking the wrists to support the bar on your forearms for the clean position, practice the motion with an unweighted bar until you get it right.

Behind-head Press. Stand with your feet about six inches apart. Legs and back should be straight. Grip your barbell so that it rests on your shoulders behind your neck. Your hands should be slightly farther apart than they were for the clean and press. Knuckles should be back. Lift the bar to full extension of the arms. Don't duck your head forward or put a sway in your back with the lift. Return the bar slowly to your shoulders and repeat.

Bends and Twists. With the barbell still on your shoulders, but feet about two feet apart, do right- and left-side bends. The weight will make this a good combination stretch-and-flex exercise. Starting from the same position, do some slow twists. Avoid any jerking motion that might swing you off balance. Twists and bends are also good warm-up exercises for weight training.

Pull-overs. Lie on your back with the barbell across your thighs. Your hands should grip the bar, knuckles up, just a few inches outside your thighs. Keeping your arms straight, lift the bar up over your head and on to the floor above your head. Let the bar touch softly and then return it slowly to the starting position and repeat.

Floor Presses. Lie on your back with your hands holding the barbell across your chest. Your knuckles should be toward your face. Cock your wrists to bring your forearms under the bar. Then straighten your arms slowly to lift the bar vertically.

DUMBBELLS

Forward and Lateral Lifts. Stand with feet together and knees straight. Hold a dumbbell in each hand, knuckles facing forward. Without bending your elbows, raise the weights forward and overhead. Lower them slowly through the same arcs. Don't let your body sway. Your shoulders should do most of the work. When the

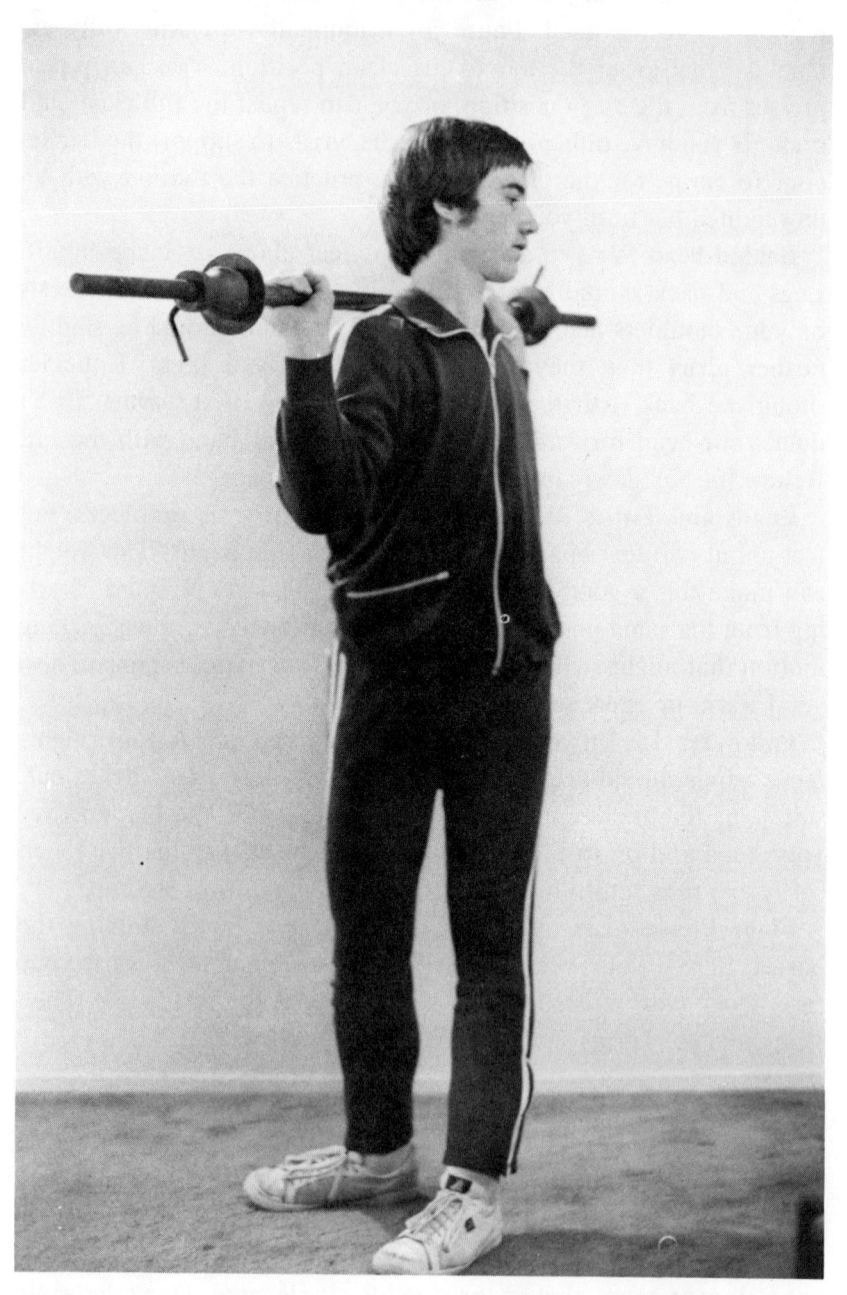

Twisting with a weight will give the lateral muscles a strong stretch. Be careful, however, to avoid overextension when twisting or bending with weights.

dumbbells are back at thigh level, turn your hands so the knuckles face outward. Now lift the weights sideways to shoulder level. Stop and turn the hands over so that your knuckles point down. Continue the lift to bring the dumbbells together overhead. Lower the weights in the same manner, stopping at shoulder level to turn them over.

Bends and Twists. Holding a dumbbell in your right hand, with both arms at your sides, do a series of side bends, left and right. Then change the dumbbell to the left hand and repeat.

With a dumbbell in each hand and arms extended sideways at shoulder level, do a series of left and right twists. Avoid a jerky motion and try to keep your arms from sagging.

Toe Lifts. With a dumbbell in each hand at thigh level, rise on your toes and then lower yourself to your heels. Do the exercise slowly. This is excellent for strengthening your ankles.

Swing Lifts. With your feet about a foot apart, straddle two dumbbells. Keeping your back straight, bend your knees to pick up a weight in each hand. Now straighten your knees vigorously and swing the weights up in an arc. Your legs should be fully straightened at about the same time the weights reach the peak overhead position. Lower the weights through the same arc, bend your knees to return the weights to the floor.

One-arm Press. Stand with your feet about a foot apart and hold a dumbbell in your right hand level with your right shoulder, knuckles toward the shoulder. Your forearm should be perpendicular beneath the weight and your elbow should be close to your right hip. Lean to the left and at the same time, lift the weight vertically with the right arm fully extended. Now straighten your body and lower the weight slowly to shoulder level, remembering to keep your forearm perpendicular. Repeat with the left arm.

Chair Press. Sitting in a chair, take a dumbbell in each hand. Hold them at your shoulders with knuckles back. Now raise them slowly overhead. When your arms are fully extended, lower the weights slowly and steadily to shoulder level. The sitting position helps hold body motion to a minimum.

Floor Press. Lie on your back with your legs straight and your feet together. Hold the dumbbells at shoulder level with knuckles

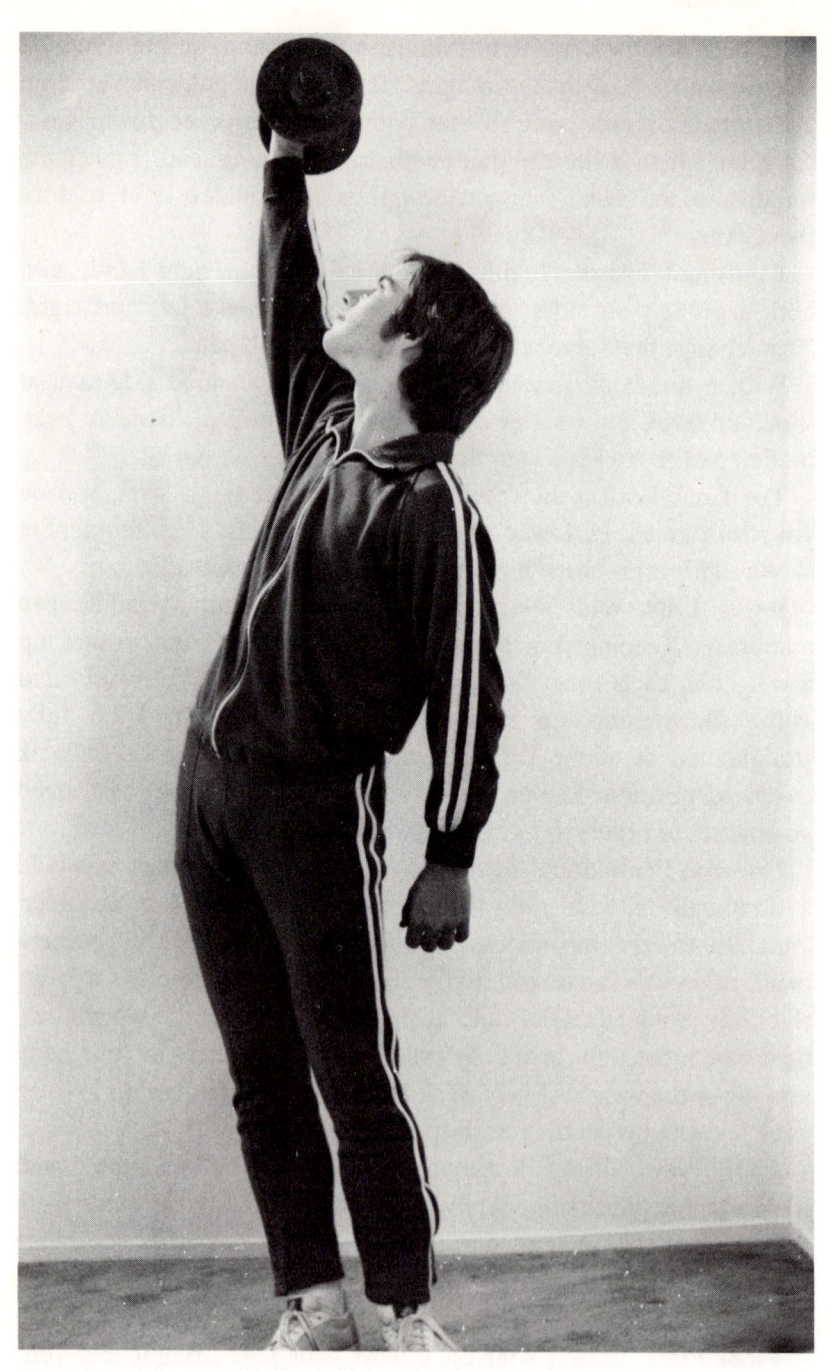

The one-arm press with a dumbbell should be done with a shift of your hips to bring them under the weight.

facing out. Lift vertically for full arm extension. Then lower slowly and repeat.

Lateral Floor Lifts. Lie on the floor with legs straight and feet together. With a dumbbell in each hand, spread your arms wide. Knuckles should face down. Without bending your elbows, lift the weights to bring them together above your chest. Lower them to the starting position slowly and repeat.

MAKING WEIGHTS

To avoid the expense of commercial weights, you can make serviceable barbells and dumbbells with broom sticks and cement-filled cans.

Cut two 18" lengths from a broomstick for your dumbbells. Drive some small nails in the sides of the sticks near each end. Set one end of each stick in pint cans and fill them with cement. Make sure the stick is centered in the can. Then let the cement cure overnight. Now place the other ends in cans and fill them with cement. Again, make sure the sticks are centered before you leave it to cure.

For barbells, the broom stick, a sturdy one with no flaws, should be 5' long. Use quart cans to mold your weights.

Homemade dumbbells and barbells provide a cheap introduction to weight training. Their major disadvantage is that you cannot increase the weight-load as you can with a set of commercial dumbbells and barbells.

As already stated, however, you should strive at first to increase repetitions rather than add weight. Later, if you feel you have advanced enough for more weight, get advice from a weight-training expert. The expert can outline an advanced program in line with your physique, telling you what your limits will be for various exercises and setting your rate of progress to reach those limits. He might also give you some good leads on where to find a set of secondhand, commercial weights.

11 *Special Problems*

Excess weight is the most common fitness problem by far in the United States. One estimate has it that half the adult population is overweight, and you sometimes get the idea that the other half is worried about the problem.

It is not a simple problem. In fact, when you are in your growing years, it is often difficult to say if you have a serious weight problem and, if so, exactly what should be done about it. You need medical advice.

Your doctor is the best judge of your body type and your development and growth, factors that are vital in any judgment of weight. Understanding these factors might relieve you right now of some unjustified worries. Let's take a brief look at them.

BODY TYPE AND GROWTH

There are three basic body types. *Endomorphs* have large, heavy bone structures. They are often taller than average and have thick, solid builds. *Ectomorphs* have light builds. They are lean, sometimes wasp-waisted with small muscles. *Mesomorphs* are stocky, often shorter than average, with thick muscles that tend to give them triangular structure.

SPECIAL PROBLEMS

You inherit your body type. No crash diet or magic pill is going to turn a large-boned *endomorph* into a wasp-waisted *ectomorph*.

If both your parents are large-boned, the chances are good that you will grow into a large-boned adult, an *endomorph*. If they have different builds, predictions are more difficult. At least, however, you should learn what to expect during growth and development.

By age five, most youngsters lose their "baby fat." They stay lean for about two years, but then bulges of "puppy fat" appear. The resulting pudginess causes little concern until puberty begins, as early as age ten for girls and age twelve for boys.

Wild things happen during puberty. These are the normal things, but they will cause worries. For one thing, both boys and girls start to worry about those bulges of "puppy fat," wondering when or if they will ever go away. They will, but for a time, fatty bulges may collect elsewhere, causing fresh worries.

The changes of puberty are touched off by a surge of chemical secretions from various glands. Body growth speeds up. In five or six years, girls will gain an average of fifty pounds and add nine inches in height. Boys will gain an average of sixty pounds and grow ten inches.

Reproduction organs develop. Girls begin menstruating and their hips widen to make room for the growth of reproductive organs, a growth that sometimes causes a temporary pot belly. For boys, the testicles descend into the scrotum, the voice changes, the shoulders broaden, and facial hair starts to grow.

The chemicals that trigger puberty have some bothersome side effects. They can make skin oily, so oily that pores become clogged and infected, causing acne. Frequent washing and other sanitary precautions are the best remedy, but even with the utmost care acne can persist, sometimes well after other signs of puberty are over.

The chemicals can also cause fatty bulges. With girls, the bulges tend to appear on the abdomen and around the hips and thighs. With boys, the fat can collect on the upper thighs, the abdomen and the nipple area of the chest.

The bulges will fade with the decline of chemical secretions. **Try not to worry about them.**

In a recent sampling of teen-age girls, 50 per cent believed they were too fat. When doctors examined them, however, it was found that just 15 per cent were overweight and, even among them, few conditions were serious.

So your doctor is the best judge of your weight problem, real or imagined. Certainly, you should have a doctor's approval before launching any drastic weight-reducing program. Even if you adopt a mild program, there are some paths you should not follow.

THINGS TO AVOID

Pills. There are three types of diet pills, and two of them can be purchased without a doctor's prescription. One is simply a sugar pill. Taking it cuts your appetite just like a candy bar between meals cuts your appetite. But the pill and the candy bar are both high in calories. You get no benefit from sugar pills, and you miss out on necessary nutriments at mealtime.

The other pill you can buy over the counter contains a chemical known as a diuretic. It makes you urinate and thus reduces body fluid and weight temporarily. This is useless. Your body must have water to function properly.

The third diet pill contains amphetamine, a drug that can cause serious side effects. It cannot be had without a prescription, and most doctors today have little faith in it. While the drug does reduce appetite at first, the effect does not last.

Sweating. Excessive sweating will reduce body fluid for a temporary weight loss, but the fluid must be replaced. Steam baths and rubberized exercise suits provide no easy short cut for reducing, and they might cause serious dehydration. Vigorous exercise, particularly during hot weather, will make you sweat, so be sure to increase your water intake to make up for the loss.

Fad Diets. Any diet that calls for unusual foods or a monotonous intake of one particular food, such as boiled cabbage or raw carrots, has to be regarded with suspicion. First of all, there is the danger of cutting yourself off from the necessary nutriments you get in a balanced diet. Secondly, you will have to be a rare person indeed to stick with one or two selected foods for more than two or

SPECIAL PROBLEMS

three weeks. True, you may lose weight during those few weeks, but what will happen when you return to your normal eating habits? The chances are that you will go back to your original weight.

Crash Diets. The same objections can be raised against diets that call for drastic reductions in food intake. Doctors may order spartan diets for patients with serious weight problems, but generally the sudden loss of weight you get from a crash diet is not considered healthy. Moderation is almost always the best guide. Most doctors will not want you to lose more than a pound a week. This calls for a slight reduction in food intake—a diet you can live with the rest of your life, and this is usually coupled with an increase in exercise. In fact, many doctors now believe that no dieting can lead to permanent weight loss if it is not done in conjunction with an exercise program.

WHAT WORKS

Remember the formula in Chapter 3: Calories equal body tissue and/or energy? This is the key to successful reducing programs. Cutting down does not mean you have to deprive yourself of all your favorite foods, but it does mean reducing your intake of high-calorie foods. Instead of that big piece of pie or cake that you've been eating for dessert, ask for a half portion. Instead of two spoonfuls of sugar in your tea or coffee, limit yourself to one spoonful. Instead of drowning your cereal in thick cream, use just half as much, or better yet, switch to skimmed milk. You can figure just what reductions must be made.

Get a calorie rating list. Many drugstores carry them. Use the list to figure how many calories you are now taking in daily. Include your snacks along with your meals, and don't forget to count the calories in soft drinks. Now multiply your body weight by fifteen to get an idea of your daily calorie requirement. The difference between the two figures will give you your target.

Suppose, for instance, that you have been consuming 2,200 calories a day, but your weight indicates a need for just 2,000 calories. You are taking in 200 calories above your budget.

As we've already seen, just a few minutes of vigorous exercise, such as jumping rope, cycling, or jogging will burn up 100 of those calories. And a slight adjustment of your eating habits will take care of the rest. That would bring your calorie equation into balance.

But you want to lose weight. You want to create a calorie deficit —using up more than you take in. Now, there are 3,500 calories stored up in a pound of body fat. To lose a pound a week, you would have to create a deficit of 500 calories a day. That would call for substantial changes in your eating habits and perhaps more exercise than you have time to fit into your daily schedule. Remember, you have already had to cut 200 calories just to bring your daily budget into balance.

So set a reasonable goal. Try for a loss of a pound every two weeks. You could create a daily deficit of 250 calories with just a little restraint at mealtime and just a little more sustained effort during the aerobic phase of your exercise program.

Stick with your new regime for six months and you will have lost twelve pounds. Perhaps that will put you at your ideal weight. If so, you can then adjust your calorie formula to do away with the deficit.

Chances are that you won't want to cut down on your exercises. That's a good sign. It means you will be able to start enjoying some of the mealtime calories you have been denying yourself. Bon appetite!

TO GAIN WEIGHT

An increase in food intake, more rest, and miometric exercises supplemented with isometrics or weight training will usually add substantial body weight.

The best single food for gaining weight is milk, but other favorites include puddings, junkets, and hot cereals. Milk-based drinks such as cocoa, malted milk, and milk shakes are also excellent. Today, there are several high-carbohydrate drinks on the market advertised as weight boosters, but they do not beat the price of whole milk.

SPECIAL PROBLEMS

An extra hour of sleep each night, and fifteen minutes of rest, preferably with the feet up, after each meal, should be part of the weight-gaining program. Meanwhile, your exercises should include lots of flexing.

Some people never seem able to gain weight no matter how hard they try. This is particularly true of active teen-agers. Their activity, combined with growth, burns up all the fuel they can take in.

Again, growth rates and body types must be considered, and ambitious weight-gaining efforts should not be undertaken without your doctor's approval. Not long ago, many young athletes were urged to gain weight to "make the team." This was particularly true of high school football. Today, however, most coaches and trainers recommend weight-gaining programs only after the athlete has been examined and given medical clearance.

LIMITATIONS

If you have a handicap that limits activity or strength, you should give particular attention to exercise. Often, exercises will help you overcome a handicap. The heroic stories of men and women who have done just that should be enough to inspire you.

Glenn Cunningham set a new world record for the mile run sixteen years after he suffered crippling burns in a fire. Patricia Neal returned to her acting career after a paralyzing stroke. Ben Hogan made a fantastic golf comeback after a devastating auto accident. The list goes on.

Of course, these are all dramatic stories that make headlines. Perhaps you have a limitation that leaves little room for change. This does not mean you should shun exercise. On the contrary, it is very important—not to make headlines but to prolong life. Far too often a phyiscal limitation is looked on as an excuse for an inactive life. This leads to poor conditioning, poor health, and sometimes increased limitations.

No matter what your handicap might be, there is certainly something you can do that will keep you in shape.

Have your doctor help you select exercises you can do. Try to include activities that will build muscle strength and keep them supple. Also, it is very important, if possible, to include an aerobic exercise of some kind.

Don't neglect sports. More and more schools and recreation departments are offering team sports and competition for the handicapped. Even people in wheelchairs compete in track and field, play basketball, and go bowling. You should be able to find some sport that will keep you active and give you pleasure.

Remember, you don't have to be on the team to make a contribution to school sports. Scorekeepers, timers, uniform and equipment managers, ticket sellers, team treasurers and secretaries, reporters, assistant trainers, and managers are always in demand.

THERAPY EXERCISES

If you ever had an illness or injury that left stiffness or weakness in a certain set of muscles, you were probably given a set of exercises to do as part of a recovery program, exercises that were prescribed by a doctor or physical therapist.

Perhaps, however, you have a weakness or minor limitation that was not caused by illness or injury. The therapy exercises can help you correct the problem. Here are some typical workouts designed for specific areas. Some, you will notice, have already been described in earlier chapters.

Shoulders and Elbows. Make a tight fist and bend your arm up and down at the elbow.

Sit on the floor beneath a low bar and do pull-ups, lifting yourself to your knees or your feet, depending on the height of the bar.

Do arm push-aways from a wall, or knee push-ups.

Holding a light weight, such as a book, in each hand, raise and lower your arms from the elbows. Then, holding the same weights, lift your arms with elbows straight both forward and to the sides.

Hands and Wrists. Make a fist repeatedly, opening and closing your hand until the fingers tire. Working with one hand, press the fingers one at a time against the thumb. With your hand open, spread the fingers wide and bring them together again. Squeeze a sponge or soft rubber ball repeatedly. Any work with the fingers, such as typing or piano playing, will strengthen them quickly.

SPECIAL PROBLEMS

With one forearm on the table and your fist clenched, bend your wrist fully both right and left. Now cock your wrist back to raise your fist while your forearm remains on the table.

You can make a wrist strengthener with a short length of broomstick, a cord, and a weight of three to five pounds. Tie one end of the cord to the weight and the other end to the middle of the broomstick. Roll the cord up on the stick with wrist action. Work with both overhand and underhand holds on the stick.

The Neck. Make circles with your head, getting maximum stretch backward, forward, and to the sides. Do this before beginning any of the neck flexing exercises. Then try standing close to a wall and pushing away with your forehead. The farther you can place your feet from the wall, the better. Next, stand with your back to the wall and push away with the back of your head. Lie on your back with knees bent and try to lift yourself to rest on your feet and your head. Lie on your stomach with a pillow under your forehead and try to lift yourself on your feet and head.

Hips, Back, and Abdomen. Sit on a chair and hold it at the sides with your hands. Keeping your head up, lean forward as far as possible and then backward. Next bend to the right and left. Now try making a full circle, bending from the hips. Still sitting hold your arms straight ahead and then twist as far as possible right and left.

Take a hands and knees position on the floor and crawl sideways to the right and then back again to the left. Lie on your back with your weight on your legs and elbows. Lift your body to put your weight on your heels and elbows. Lie on your back with arms across your chest. Lift your head and shoulders off the floor. Lie on your stomach and arch your back to lift shoulders and legs off the floor. You can use your arms to lift your shoulders at first, but eventually you will want to do this on the strength of lower back alone.

Feet, Ankles, and Knees. Work at picking up small stones or marbles with your toes. Sitting on a chair, rock your feet up and down on the floor from toes to heels. Try for maximum flex and extension. In the same position, lift your legs off the floor and make circles with your feet. Put a board or stack of magazines on the floor two to three inches high. Stand with your heels on the floor and the balls of your feet on the platform. Lift yourself on your toes, then lower to your heels slowly. Hold weights in your hands to increase the flex.

BALANCE AND CO-ORDINATION

Don't get the idea that you can do nothing to improve balance and co-ordination. You can develop them with exercise just as you can develop strength and flexibility. Many of the exercises already covered in earlier chapters, such as jumping jacks, upside-down bicycles, and several Yoga exercises have been singled out for balance and co-ordination benefits.

Here are some other things you can try.

For Better Balance. Stand with your feet together for a ten-second count. Now close your eyes and count another ten seconds. When you can do this without letting your body sway, advance to

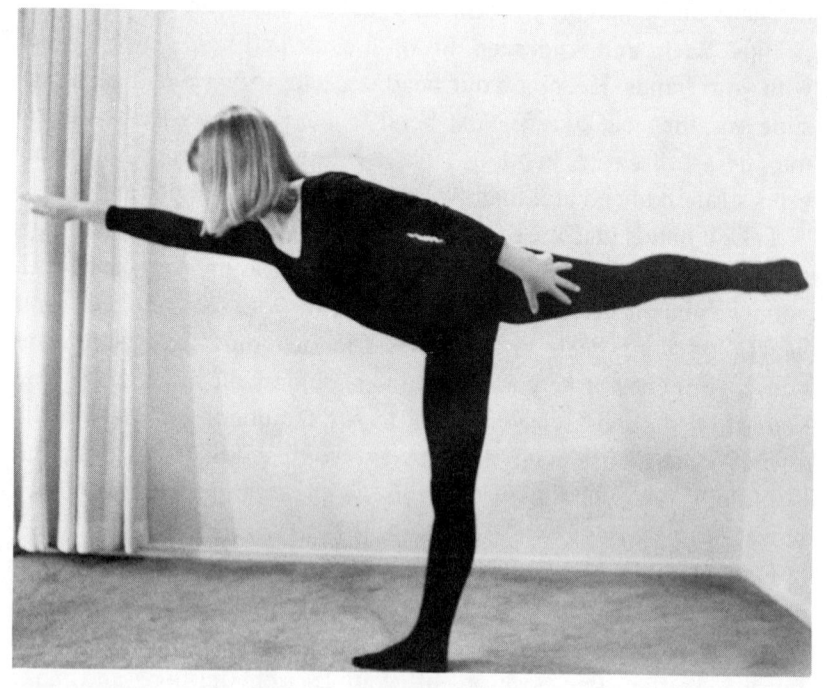

This ballet pose will develop balance and grace. Don't get the idea it's just for girls. Boys often need balance training more than girls. You can begin with the extended hand on a chair.

SPECIAL PROBLEMS

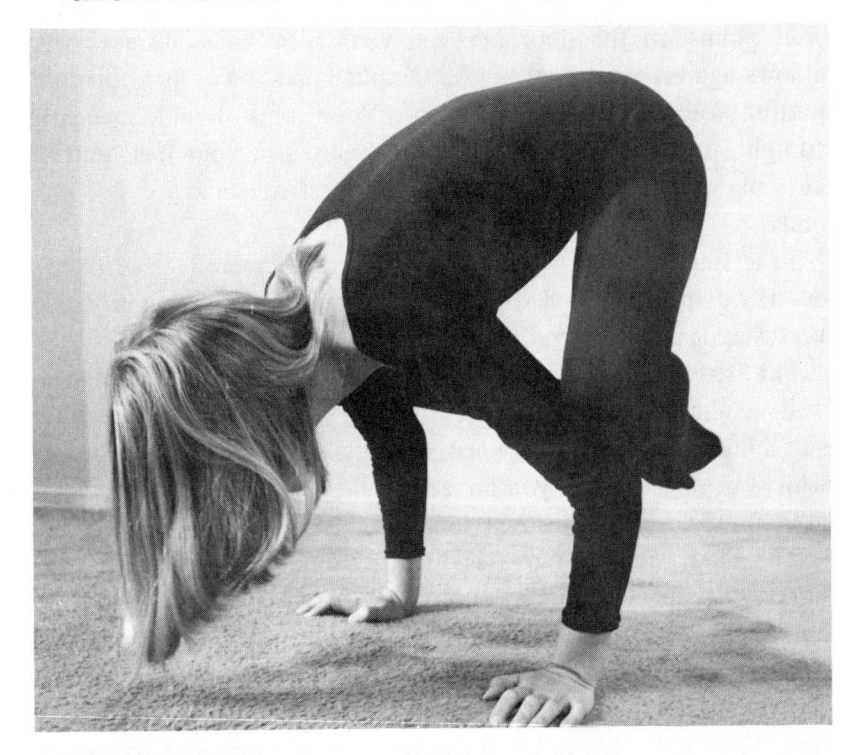

Frog stand.

foot lifts. Keeping your eyes closed, lift one foot ten inches off the floor and hold the position for ten seconds. Repeat with the other foot raised.

Now, with your eyes open, try a ballet pose. Standing on one leg, lift the other leg backward as you lean forward with your body. Your raised leg and your body should make a line parallel to the floor. Hold for ten seconds. If this is too difficult, begin with your hands braced on a chairback. Keep working until you can hold the position on either leg for ten seconds without any support. Now see if you can do it with your eyes closed. If you can, you have developed excellent body balance.

To improve posture as well as balance, try walking with a book on your head. Walk a straight line. Do some half knee bends. Try some slow body twists. Dancers in training go through a whole series of motions with a book balanced on their heads.

Frog stands look more difficult than they actually are. Squat with your palms on the floor between your bent knees. Brace your elbows against your thighs close to your knees. Now lean forward, putting your weight on your arms. Your arms should be nearly straight, pressing against your inner thighs. Lift your feet, putting all your weight on your arms. Hold your frog stand for five seconds.

Frog stands will give you confidence to advance to head stands described in Chapter 8 and, as suggested, you can begin doing head stands against a wall.

For Better Co-ordination. Toe taps will stimulate circulation as well as sharpen co-ordination. Standing with your arms at your sides, jump and bring your knees up quickly, trying to tap your feet with your fingers while you are still in the air. If this is too difficult at first, tap a hand on just one foot.

The loop walk is a real challenge. Bend over and lace your fingers together, making a loop of your arms. Stretch to get your hands as low as possible. Now step through the loop one foot at a time so that your hands end up behind your calves. Next, step back one foot at a time to the starting position. If this is too difficult at first, hold a broomstick with your hands about shoulder-width apart. Step over the broomstick. The loop walk develops both balance and co-ordination. At the same time it gives those shoulder and arm muscles a good stretch. It's another good all-around exercise.

FINAL WORDS

They say that habits formed early last a lifetime. I hope that exercise becomes an early habit for you, and that hope, as you must know by now, is the same thing as wishing you a long and happy life.

Index

Abdomen, 71–74, 116–17
  lean-aways, 116, 117
  muscles, strengthening, 4–5
  pull-ins, 116–17
  rocking V's, 73–74
  sit-ups, 71–72
  twisting sit-ups, 72–73
Acid tolerance, increasing, 25
Advanced leg pulls, 102
Advanced push-ups, 79
Aerobics, 83–95
  books on, 94–95
  jogging and running, 89–92
  meaning of, 14
  muscle size and, 24–25
  skipping rope, 86–88
  sports, 94
  stationary running, 9–10, 85–86
  swimming, 92–93
  walking, 89
Aerobics (Cooper), 94
Air pollution, lung capacity and, 21
Alternate leg pulls, 104–5
Alveoli, 20
Amino acids, 30, 31
Anaerobic ("without oxygen")
    exercises, 25
Ankle lifts, 81, 82
Arching, 54
Arm pulls, 123
Arm pushes, 123–24
Arms and chest, 77–81, 122–24
  arm pulls, 123

  arm pushes, 123–24
  hand lifts, 122
Arms, neck, and shoulders, 56–60
  arm swings, 58–60
  hand waggles, 57–58
  head rotations, 56
  pumps, 60
Arm swings, 58–60

Back, 74–76, 100–4
  bow, 101–3
  leg pull, 100–1
  leg raises, 74–75
  leg and trunk lifts, 75–76
  leg whips, 75
  plow, 103–4
  spreads and flutters, 76
  twist, 103
  Yoga bend, 100
Back bend, 108, 109
Back kicks, 68
Balance and co-ordination, 144–46
  for better balance, 144–46
  for better co-ordination, 146
Ballet pose, 144
Barbell exercises, 128–31
  behind-head press, 131
  bends and twists, 131
  clean and press, 128–131
  floor presses, 131
  pull-overs, 131
  snatch, 128
  two-hand curl, 128

INDEX

Basic training (U. S. Army), 13
Basketball, 94
Beer and wine, 36
Behind-head press (with a barbell), 131
Bend, the, 1–3
   back exercise, 108, 109
Bends, 61–62
Bends and twists (with a barbell), 131
Bends and twists (with dumbbells), 133
Blood circulation, 21–22, 25
Body control, 12–13
Body lifts, 76
Body measurements, taking, 45–46
Body talk, 17–46
   body system, 19–27
   food for fitness, 28–36
   physical-fitness test, 37–46
Body type and growth, 136–38
Bow, 101–3
Breads and cereal (food) group, 35–36
Breathers, taking, 4, 7–9
Bridge, the, 105
Buck chins, 92

Calcium, 34
Calisthenics, 13, 14
Calories, 29–30
Carbohydrates, 31
Carbon, 30, 31
Carbon monoxide, 21
Cells, body, 19–20, 25
Chair press (with dumbbells), 133
Chest and arms, 77–81, 122–24
   advanced push-ups, 79
   elbow push-ups, 78–79
   pull-ups, 79–81
   push-up training, 77–78
   See also Arms, neck, and shoulders
Chest cavity, expansion and contraction of, 21
Cholesterol, 32
Cigarette smokers, 21
Circulatory system, 21–22, 25
Clean and press (with a barbell), 128–31
Cobra, the, 3
Cooling off, 10
Cooper, Dr. Kenneth H., 14, 21, 83, 84, 85, 86, 91, 93, 94, 115
Crash diets, avoiding, 139
Crawl, the, 59
Cycling, 93

Dairy products, 34
Dehydration, 29

Diet pills, 138
Diets, what to avoid, 138–39
Double leg lifts, 65–66
Double leg overs, 67
Dumbbells, 131–35
   bends and twists, 133
   chair press, 133
   floor press, 133–34
   forward and lateral lifts, 131–33
   lateral floor lifts, 135
   one-arm press, 133, 134
   swing lifts, 133
   toe lifts, 133

Ectomorph (body type), 136, 137
Elbow pumps, 60
Elbow push-ups, 78–79
Endomorph (body type), 136, 137
Excess fat, 26–27
Exercise
   aerobics, 83–95
   and body talk, 17–46
   common sense about, vii
   introduction to, 1–15
   isometrics, 115–26
   miometrics, 70–82
   pliometrics, 25, 49–69
   special problems, 136–46
   supplementals, 97–135
   weights, 127–35
   Yoga, 3, 99–114
   See also types of exercise

Fad diets, avoiding, 138–39
Fats, 31–32
   saturated and unsaturated, 32
Fat tissue, 26–27
Feet, ankles, and knees therapy, 143–44
Flexing, 4–6
   push-ups, 5–6, 7
   sit-ups, 4–5
   taking a breather, 7–9
Floor press (with a barbell), 131
Floor press (with dumbbells), 133–34
Flutters, *see* Spreads and flutters
Foods, 28–36
   bread and cereal, 35–36
   calories, 29–30
   carbohydrates, 31
   categories of, 34–36
   fats, 31–32
   fruit and vegetables, 35
   junk, 36
   meat, 35
   milk, 34, 140
   proteins, 30–31

INDEX

vitamins, 32–34
water, 28–29
Foot presses, 120–21
Forward and lateral lifts (with dumbbells), 131–33
Frog stands, 145–46
Fructose, 31
Fruit and vegetable (food) group, 35

Galactose, 31
Glucose, 31
Glycerol, 31
Golf, 94
Grace and balance, 111–12, 113
Gross, Leonard, 95

Half lotus position, 110
Handball, 94
Hand lifts, 122
Hands and wrists therapy, 142–43
Hand waggles, 57–58
Head presses, 124–25
Head rotations, 56
Head stands, 111–12
Heart and circulatory ailments, 21
Heart beat, 22
Heart rate (or pulse), 22–24
  taking your own, 23–24
Hips, back, and abdomen therapy, 143
Hockey, 94
Hurdler's stretch, 67–68
Hydrogen, 30, 31

Injury, therapy exercises, 142–44
Iodine, 34
Iron, 34
Isometrics, 115–26
  abdomen, 116–17
  arms and chest, 112–24
  legs and hips, 117–21
  meaning of, 14
  neck and back, 124–25

Jogging and running, 21, 22, 89–92; see also Stationary running
Jumping jacks, 69
Jump Rope! (Skolnik), 88
Junk foods, 36

Knee bends, 82
Knee presses, 119–20
Knee pulls, 62–64
Knee pushes, 117–19
Knee push-ups, 6
Kraus, Dr. Hans, 38
Kraus-Weber Test, 38–39, 41

Lacrosse, 94
Lactic acid, athletes and, 25–26
Lateral floor lifts (with dumbbells), 135
Lateral muscles, 76–77
  body lifts, 76
  leg extensions, 76–77
  two-leg lift, 76
Lean-aways, 116, 117
Leg and arm raise, 112
Leg and trunk lifts, 75–76
Leg extensions, 76–77
Leg pull, 100–1
  advanced, 102
  alternate, 104–5
Leg raises, 74–75
Legs, 61–69, 82, 104–9, 110
  alternate pulls, 104–5
  ankle lifts, 81, 82
  back bend, 108, 109
  back kicks, 68
  bends, 61–62
  bridge, 105
  double lifts, 65–66
  double overs, 67
  half lotus position, 110
  hurdler's stretch, 67–68
  jumping jacks, 69
  knee bends, 82
  knee pulls, 62–64
  lotus position, 109, 110
  pick, the, 62, 63
  scissors, 68
  single lift, 64–65
  single overs, 66
  thigh stretch, 106–8
  thigh stretcher, 68–69
  toe twist, 105–6, 107
  upside-down bicycles, 10–12, 82
Legs and hips, 117–21
  foot presses, 120–21
  knee presses, 119–20
  knee pushes, 117–19
  tight seat, 117
Leg whips, 75
Ligaments and tendons, 26
Loop walk, 146
Lotus position, 109, 110
Lungs, 20–21

Meat (food) group, 35
Mesomorph (body type), 136
Metabolism, 27
Milk, 34, 140
Minerals, 34
Miometrics, 70–82
  abdomen, 71–74

back, 74–76
chest and arms, 77–81
lateral muscles, 76–77
legs, 82
meaning of, 14
Morehouse, Dr. Laurence E., 95
Muscle pulls, 26
Muscles, 24–26
abdominal, strengthening, 4–5
disuse of, 12–13
lactic-acid build-up in, 25–26
skeletal, 24
smooth, 24
soreness, 26
Muscle tissue cells, 19

Neck and back, 124–25
head presses, 124–25
sitting lifts, 125
Neck and shoulders, 110–11
neck twist, 111
shoulder raise, 110–11
Neck therapy, 143
Neck twist, 111
New Aerobics, The (Cooper), 94
Nitrogen, 30

One-arm press (with dumbbells), 133, 134
Oxygen, 20, 21, 30, 31, 83–84

Phosphorus, 34
Physical fitness, *see* Body control
Physical-fitness test, 37–46
keeping a record, 45–46
Kraus-Weber Test, 38–39
Youth Fitness Test, 39–45
Pick, the, 62, 63
Pills, avoiding, 138
Pliometrics, 25, 49–69
arms, neck, and shoulders, 56–60
legs, 61–69
meaning of, 14
trunk, 50–54
Plow, the, 103–4
President's Council on Physical Fitness, 39
Progress, measuring, 7–8
Proteins, 30–31
Pull-ins, 116–17
Pull-overs (with a barbell), 131
Pull-ups, 79–81
on a high bar, 80
Pull-ups (Youth Fitness Test)
for boys, 39
for girls, 39–41
Pulse, 22–24
taking your own, 23–24

Pumps, elbow, 60
Push-aways (from the wall), 7
Push-ups, 5–6, 7
advanced, 79
conventional, 5–6
elbow, 78–79
knee, 6
preparation for, 7
Push-up training, 77–78

Reaching, 50–52
and muscle strength, 51
Red blood cells, 21–22
Respiratory system, 20–21
Rocking V's, 73–74
Rope, skipping, 86–88
Rotations
head, 56
trunk, 54
Roughage, 24
Rowing, 94
Running, *see* Jogging and running; Stationary running

Saturated fats, 32
Scissors, 68
Shin splints (or buck shins), 92
Shoulder raise, 110–11
Shoulders and elbows therapy, 142
Shoulder stand, 112
Shuttle run, test for physical fitness, 42–43
Side bends, 111
Single leg lift, 64–65
Single leg overs, 66
Sitting lifts, 125
Sit-ups, 4–5, 8, 71–72
test for physical fitness, 41
twisting, 72–73
Six-hundred-yard time, test for physical fitness, 44–45
Skeletal muscles, 24
Skipping rope, 86–88
Skolnik, Peter L., 88
Smooth muscles, 24
Snatch (with a barbell), 128
Soccer, 94
Soreness, muscle, 26
Spasms, 26
Special problems, 136–46
balance and co-ordination, 144–46
body type and growth, 136–38
to gain weight, 140–41
key to success, 139–40
limitations, 141–42
therapy exercises, 142–44
things to avoid, 138–39
Sports, 94

INDEX

Spreads and flutters, 76
Sprints, 25
  test for physical fitness, 43
Squash, 94
Standing broad jump, test for physical fitness, 41–42
Stationary running, 9–10, 85–86; *see also* Jogging and running
Stretching, 1–3, 25
  bend, 1–3
  cobra, 3
  taking a breather, 4
  See also Yoga
Substitution, 8
Swaying, 52–54
Sweating, avoiding, 138
Swimming, 92–93
Swing lifts (with dumbbells), 133

Tendons, 26
Tension, reducing, 25
Therapy, 142–44
  feet, ankles, and knees, 143–44
  hands and wrists, 142–43
  hips, back, and abdomen, 143
  neck, 143
  shoulders and elbows, 142
Thigh stretch, 106–8
Thigh stretcher, 68–69
Throwing power, test for physical fitness, 43–44
Tight seat, 117
Tobacco smoking, 21
Toe lifts (with dumbbells), 133
Toe twist, 105–6, 107
Total Fitness (Morehouse and Gross), 95
Trunk, 50–54
  arching, 54
  leg and trunk lifts, 75–76
  reaching, 50–52
  rotations, 54
  swaying, 52–54
  twisting, 54
Twist, the, 103
Twisting, 54, 55
  with a weight, 132
Twisting sit-ups, 72–73
Two-hand curl (with a barbell), 128
Two-leg lift, 76

United States Air Force, 14, 83
United States Department of Agriculture (USDA), 28, 34, 35, 36
Unsaturated fats, 32
Upside-down bicycle, 10–12, 82

Vegetarians, 31
Vital capacity, 21
Vitamin A, 33, 34
Vitamin B_1, 33, 35
Vitamin B_2, 33, 34, 35
Vitamin B_3, 33
Vitamin B_6, 33
Vitamin B_{12}, 33
Vitamin C, 33, 34, 35
Vitamin D, 33, 34
Vitamin E, 33–34
Vitamin K, 33
Vitamins, 32–34

Walking, 89
Wall push-aways, 7
Warm-up exercises, importance of, 26
Water, 28–29
Weber, Dr. Sonja, 38
Weight, gaining, 140–41
Weights, 127–35
  barbell exercises, 128–31
  dumbbells, 131–35
  making your own, 135
Weight training, 14–15
White blood cells, 21
World War I, 13

Yoga, 3, 99–114
  back, 100–4
  grace and balance, 111–12, 113
  legs, 104–9, 110
  meaning of, 14
  neck and shoulders, 110–11
Yoga bend, 100
Youth Fitness Test, 39–45
  pull-ups for boys, 39
  pull-ups for girls, 39–41
  shuttle run, 42–43
  sit-ups, 41
  six-hundred-yard time, 44–45
  sprint, 43
  standing broad jump, 41–42

Although born in Los Angeles, RICHARD B. LYTTLE is really a product of rural California. He graduated from high school in Ojai, served in the Navy in the 1940s, and attended the University of California at Berkeley, where he majored in English and professed boxing as his sport. He graduated with a B.A. degree and several bruises.

Mr. Lyttle worked as a cowboy, farmer, newspaper reporter, editor, bartender, and school bus driver. He began selling stories and articles for children in the 1950s. He sold more than 150 articles before turning to books. This is his thirteenth book.

The author has retained an interest in sports, particularly sailing, tennis, track and field, bicycling, and baseball. He is an enthusiastic camper and trout fisherman.

Mr. Lyttle, his wife, Jean, and their children live in a small town north of San Francisco, and next-door to the Point Reyes National Seashore.